The Women's Concise Guide to a Healthier Heart

THE WOMEN'S
CONCISE GUIDE TO
A HEALTHIER
HEART

Karen J. Carlson, M.D.

Stephanie A. Eisenstat, M.D.

Terra Ziporyn, Ph.D.

Harvard University Press
Cambridge, Massachusetts
London, England · 1997

Library of Congress Cataloging-in-Publication Data

Carlson, Karen J.
The women's concise guide to a healthier heart /
Karen J. Carlson, Stephanie A. Eisenstat, Terra Ziporyn.
p.   cm.
Includes bibliographical references and index.
ISBN 0-674-95483-1 (cloth). — ISBN 0-674-95484-X (paper)
1. Heart—Diseases.   2. Women—Diseases.   3. Heart—Diseases—Sex factors.
I. Eisenstat, Stephanie A.   II. Ziporyn, Terra Diane, 1958–   .   III. Title.
RC682.C44   1997
616.1′2′0082—dc21   97-17310

*Illustrations by Harriet Greenfield on pages 10, 14, 15, 19, 24, 25,
30, 33, 35, 36, 37, 39, 47, 49, 51, 56, 68, 69, 85, 102.
Illustrations by Susan Keller on pages 79, 94.*

Contents

The Women's Concise Guide
to a Healthier Heart

Introduction

There is a slow-dying myth that heart disease is a problem from which women are somehow exempt. This myth flies in the face of the reality that 2.5 million American women are hospitalized annually for heart disease. Approximately 500,000 American women die of heart problems each year, half of them because of coronary artery disease. In fact, coronary artery disease is the most frequent cause of death among women in the United States. On top of that, at least 300,000 American women, most of whom are of childbearing age, have a congenital malformation of the cardiovascular system.

Despite these statistics, astoundingly little research has been conducted on the best ways to diagnose, treat, and prevent heart disease in women. Nor have there been extensive studies of the different psychological, social, or economic factors that may bear on the way heart disease affects women. Until quite recently most studies of heart disease involved only men. Women of childbearing age were excluded because researchers claimed that compounding variables such as menstrual cycle changes would only complicate results. And older women were excluded because they tended to have more coexisting illnesses than men. What these studies failed to address was that these very "confounding" factors might have some bearing on how heart disease manifests itself in women and on the methods that might work in preventing and treating it. Studies under way today are attempting to take the other variables into account.

Heart disease, also called cardiovascular disease, includes a myriad of disorders involving the heart and its blood vessels. Many of these fall into the category of coronary heart disease, a term that itself encompasses a variety of conditions. Most coronary heart disease is due to a process known as atherosclerosis, in which fat and cholesterol are deposited in the inner walls of arteries throughout the body. Over the years, scar tissue and other debris build up as more fat and cholesterol are deposited. If one or more of the arteries that

1

supply the heart muscle with blood are seriously narrowed (a condition called coronary artery disease), and especially if a blood clot forms at a site of the narrowing, the heart cannot get enough oxygen from the bloodstream. The result is chest pain (angina pectoris)— and possibly a heart attack.

In addition to coronary artery disease and angina pectoris, coronary heart disease includes other disorders that may be complications of atherosclerosis, including congestive heart failure and arrhythmias. Women are also likely to encounter several problems of the heart valves that are not (or are not always) caused by atherosclerosis. All of these heart conditions are described in the following pages of this book.

Many of the risk factors for cardiovascular disease are thought to be similar in both sexes—obesity, cigarette smoking, hypertension, diabetes, a sedentary lifestyle, a family history of heart disease, and possibly stress, high blood cholesterol, and high blood fat levels. Other major differences between the sexes do exist when it comes to the heart. These differences are biological, medical, and social.

Biological differences between the sexes. The rate of coronary heart disease is low in women during the reproductive years. Only 1 in 1,000 women aged 35 to 44 and 4 in 1,000 women aged 45 to 54 can expect to develop coronary heart disease. (These statistics are true for all women except diabetic women, who are at highest risk of all groups.)

After menopause women's risk of cardiovascular disease rises by a factor of 2 or 3. Surgical removal of both ovaries before natural menopause occurs can increase the risk of having a heart attack by a factor of 3. The increased risk after menopause is usually attributed to a decrease in estrogen production; estrogen protects the coronary arteries from the onset of atherosclerosis.

Although cardiovascular disease tends to develop later in life in women than in men, it is more likely to be fatal once it does develop. Women with heart disease are twice as likely as men to die within 2 months of their first heart attack and are more likely to suffer a second heart attack.

The biological reasons for these differences have not been well studied, but it is known that both the heart and the coronary arteries in women are smaller and lighter than those of men, and this may have some effect on the atherosclerotic process or on the response to treatment. An added factor is that women with heart disease (because they are generally older than men when it develops) tend to have other systemic diseases at the same time.

Medications and operations that work well for men are not always as successful in women. For example, thrombolytic therapy, which involves administering clot-busting drugs to treat heart attacks, works just as well in women as in men at dissolving life-threatening blood clots. Women, however, more frequently develop serious bleeding complications after taking these drugs. In addition, because many women's heart attacks are more severe, because they have other health problems, and because they are older on average than men who have heart attacks, they are less likely to be good candidates for this therapy in the first place.

Surgical procedures to treat coronary heart disease—such as balloon angioplasty (which stretches the arteries with an inflatable balloon), coronary atherectomy (in which atherosclerotic plaques are removed from the arteries), and coronary bypass surgery (in which detours are built around blocked arteries)—are not offered to women as frequently as to men, partly because they simply do not work as well in women. Although long-term survival after these operations seems to be comparable in both sexes, women tend to experience more complications following surgery and are twice as likely as men to continue having symptoms of their disease 4 years after coronary angioplasty.

It is still not clear whether various medications, including aspirin, beta blockers, and calcium-channel blockers, have the same efficacy in both men and women, at least for all applications. Lipid (blood fat) lowering drugs (including Mevacor and Lopid) have not been adequately studied in women either, particularly in the women most likely to be using them—those past the age of 60.

Medical differences between the sexes. Heart disease is not diagnosed until later stages in women, in part because both clinicians and women themselves are less apt to recognize symptoms for what they are. In contrast with the chest pain that men tend to experience, women's symptoms of heart disease may be vague: dull chest pressure, shortness of breath, upset stomach, persistent heartburn, weakness or fatigue. Even when women have chest pain, in most medical centers they are much less likely than men with similar symptoms to receive tests such as a stress electrocardiogram, which determines how well the heart performs during exercise. When women are given stress tests, their hearts seem to respond differently to exercise than men's and give different readings. As a result, it is sometimes difficult to interpret abnormalities in a woman's ECG according to standards established in studies of men.

Women are also less likely to be referred for coronary angiography, which can show blockage of coronary arteries. They receive fewer invasive surgeries and cardiac medications than men with similar or less severe symptoms. In addition, women are referred less frequently to rehabilitation centers, enroll less frequently, and have poorer attendance than men, possibly because relatively few rehabilitation programs have been developed that pay special attention to the exercise abilities and psychosocial needs of older women.

Whether all of this means that women are receiving too little care, men are receiving too much, or both are getting appropriate amounts remains to be determined.

Social differences between the sexes. Another part of the answer to why the course of heart disease is different in men and women may lie in social factors. Older women (who tend to be the ones who develop cardiovascular disease) may be less likely than men of the same age to have a spouse who pushes them to seek care or who helps them with household duties once they have returned from the hospital. This may in part explain why women who are referred to cardiac rehabilitation programs tend to go much less frequently than men.

Women are more likely than men to suffer from anxiety and depression after they have had a heart attack or surgery for CAD. Some investigators have postulated that these psychological symptoms may be related to the fact that women who have had heart attacks tend to be relatively sicker than their male counterparts and less able to resume normal activities. Women seem to take longer than men to recover from heart attacks and lose more days of work because of heart symptoms in general. Women also return to paid employment after a heart attack less often than do men.

Because depression and anxiety disorders are very common in

women, sometimes women experiencing chest pain and rapid heart-beat are incorrectly assumed not to have coexisting cardiovascular disease. In fact, depression and panic disorders can complicate heart disease further and increase the mortality risk. Women who are taking psychotropic drugs for the treatment of depression or anxiety should mention this fact to their clinician. Not only can many of these drugs have effects on the heart, but certain heart medications (such as beta blockers) can have psychiatric effects as well.

Women with cardiovascular disease also need to speak up about work and family responsibilities that may interfere with their treatment plans. If necessary they may discuss ways to juggle these tasks with a clinician, psychologist, or socialworker, so that outside responsibilities do not jeopardize their health and well-being.

Heart Disease
in Women

Angina Pectoris

Angina pectoris literally means pain in the chest. It generally occurs in self-limited attacks (10 or 15 minutes at most), which can be triggered by anything that increases the heart's workload and its need for blood and oxygen beyond its capacity. This includes such everyday exertions as walking, lifting groceries, and shoveling snow, emotional stress, exposure to cold, or even eating a heavy meal. Pain occurs because of an imbalance between increased demand for blood and oxygen to the heart muscle and inadequate supply, a condition called myocardial ischemia.

Although angina is not always a precursor to a heart attack, even occasional attacks of angina can be a sign of serious coronary artery disease and should be called to the attention of a physician. *Any woman who experiences a heavy squeezing pain or pressure across her chest that lasts longer than 20 minutes should seek emergency care immediately. She may be having a life-threatening heart attack.*

▸ Who is likely to develop angina?

Before the age of 75 men are more likely to have angina than women. The prevalence of angina in women increases with age, however, so that after the age of 75 angina is more common among women. Angina in women often takes a somewhat different course. Although most angina in both sexes is brought on by physical exertion, more women than men experience angina after emotional stress—or even during sleep or rest.

One explanation for this difference is that most angina in men is due to atherosclerosis—a process in which the arteries become clogged with fatty plaque. When this condition develops in the arteries of the heart, it is called coronary artery disease (CAD), and it can lead to heart attack if untreated. Angina in women under 50 may be due either to atherosclerosis or to spasms of the arteries supplying the heart (see illustration). Spasm is a sudden but tem-

Two causes of angina in women

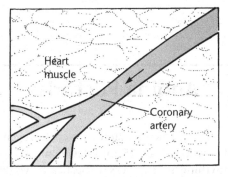

Normal flow of blood to heart muscle

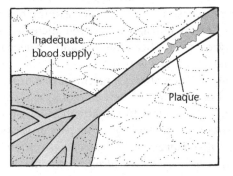

Atherosclerosis, leading to blockage of the artery, inadequate blood flow to heart muscle, and therefore chest pain

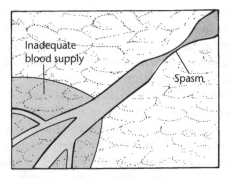

Cardiac spasm, also leading to inadequate blood flow to heart muscle and chest pain

porary narrowing of the layer of smooth muscle inside coronary arteries that helps regulate blood flow. This kind of angina, characterized by pain during rest, is called variant angina, Prinzmetal's angina, or rest angina. Its prevalence in women helps explain why some younger women, whose arteries are free of coronary artery disease, still experience angina. Variant angina seems to result in serious complications or death less often than does more typical angina. In fact, 90 percent of people with this form of angina can expect to be alive 5 years after diagnosis.

No one fully understands just what triggers coronary artery spasm. Various factors are under investigation. These include overzealous platelets (blood components responsible for clotting), cigarette smoking, and stress. Whatever the ultimate cause, all spasm is preceded by an influx of the mineral calcium into the smooth muscle cells that line the arteries.

Other women with symptoms of angina may have a condition called microvascular angina (formerly called syndrome X). Although many people with this syndrome, most of whom are women, have characteristic abnormalities in their electrocardiogram (ECG), they often have unblocked coronary arteries and normal heart function and rarely show any signs of oxygen deprivation to the heart during exercise or stress. Some researchers suspect that microvascular angina may be due to some dysfunction of tiny arteries near the larger coronary arteries.

Although these variations in women are more common under the age of 50, most women over 50 with angina have typical angina—the same type that men have—and it is caused by atherosclerosis and coronary artery disease. CAD is the most frequent cause of death among women in the United States.

Women rarely develop atherosclerosis before their late 50s or 60s; men under the age of 60 are generally more likely than women to develop this condition. The increase in atherosclerosis in women in their late 50s is related in part to lower levels of estrogen, which declines after menopause. But women under 60 who have diabetes or high blood pressure seem to be at higher risk than their male counterparts, and having a close relative with atherosclerosis also increases the odds that a woman will develop this problem. In both sexes, smoking cigarettes raises the risk of atherosclerosis, as does a sedentary lifestyle.

Variant angina and microvascular angina are more likely to occur at younger ages. Microvascular angina sometimes occurs in women near or just past menopause—suggesting that it might somehow be linked to falling estrogen levels. A few women with variant angina seem to have other conditions involving arterial spasm, such as migraine headaches, Raynaud's phenomenon (a condition in which fingers or toes turn temporarily white and blue after exposure to cold or sometimes after emotional stress), and, occasionally, aspirin-induced asthma. Many are also heavy cigarette smokers, and it is possible that smoking causes arteries to go into spasm.

▸ What are the symptoms?

Angina is itself a symptom rather than a unique disorder. It is often described as a tight, band-like, suffocating, or crushing sensation in the chest, which may radiate to the throat, shoulder, jaw, neck, or either arm. Attacks of typical angina are brought on by exercise or emotional stress, generally last only a few minutes, and are relieved by rest. If pain lasts longer than about 20 minutes, a clinician should be consulted because of the possibility of long-term damage to the heart. With medications, angina can be controlled and the risk of heart attack diminished.

The pain of variant angina or microvascular angina is often indistinguishable from that of typical angina. Variant angina often occurs in frequent spurts, however, followed by long pain-free periods.

▸ How is the condition evaluated?

Women with chest pain far too often fail to be evaluated for angina or for coronary artery disease in general. Although the likelihood of typical angina is quite low in a premenopausal woman, any woman with symptoms suggesting this problem should at the very least speak to her clinician about her personal risk factors for cardiovascular disease. If the chest pain is suggestive of angina, she should probably have an electrocardiogram done both during rest and after exercise to see if the heart muscle shows signs of damage or diminished blood flow that threatens future damage. If findings are normal, the clinician will look for causes of the pain other than heart disease.

Chest pain similar to that of a heart attack or angina is sometimes due to a totally unrelated condition called pericarditis. This inflammation of the membranous sac surrounding the heart muscle is equally common in both sexes but is more common in younger people. Pericarditis is often due to a viral infection, and frequently begins with a cold (upper respiratory tract infection). It can also result from the viruses that cause mumps, influenza, mononucleosis, chicken pox, rubella (German measles), and hepatitis B.

Viral pericarditis, while often dramatic and quite painful, is usually not a serious condition. It disappears on its own after 1 to 3 weeks, and pain can usually be relieved with aspirin or other mild analgesics. But because the symptoms of pericarditis are so similar to that of a heart attack (except that moving the chest rarely exacerbates heart attack pain), anyone who suspects she has pericarditis needs to see a physician immediately. The two conditions can be differentiated by means of blood tests, a physical examination, and an electrocardiogram.

In older women, or in women who have abnormal ECGs, further tests may be done, including echocardiography, stress testing with or without nuclear imaging, cardiac catheterization with coronary arteriography, or pharmacological stress testing (administration of various drugs that challenge the heart and other muscles; for all of these procedures see Coronary Artery Disease).

▸ How is angina treated?

Until more studies focused specifically on women are done, women with otherwise uncontrollable angina should continue to use the same drugs as men. Among the most effective and best tolerated are nitrates, beta blockers, and calcium-channel blockers. Just which drug is appropriate can vary according to a woman's overall health.

Nitroglycerin. Traditionally angina has been treated simply and quickly by placing a tablet of nitroglycerin under the tongue. This drug and other nitrates, which dilate (widen) coronary arteries and increase blood flow to the heart, are also available in the form of a spray as well as ointments, slow-release patches that can be applied directly to the skin, and oral pills.

Beta blockers. This class of drugs lowers blood pressure and stabilizes heartbeat, allowing more time for the partially obstructed coronary arteries to fill with blood. These now classic medications have

How the body's natural wound healing can cause a heart attack

NORMAL CORONARY ARTERY

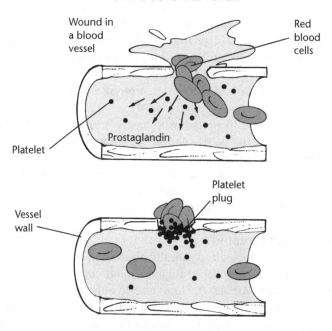

Wound in a blood vessel

Red blood cells

Platelet

Prostaglandin

Platelet plug

Vessel wall

When a blood vessel wall is injured, platelets normally help stop the bleeding by collecting at the site. They emit messengers, including prostaglandins, which summon other cells to repair the damaged vessel. As a result, oxygen-carrying red blood cells continue to move through the artery to nourish vital organs such as the heart.

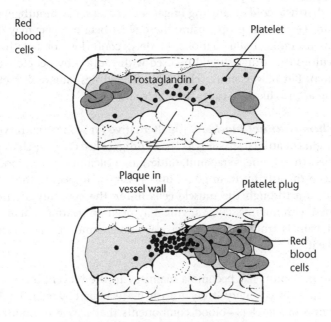

ATHEROSCLEROTIC CORONARY ARTERY

Red blood cells

Platelet

Prostaglandin

Plaque in vessel wall

Platelet plug

Red blood cells

Platelets can also collect at the site of an atherosclerotic plaque that already partially blocks a coronary artery. This normally protective response to injury in the vessel wall can stop the flow of red blood cells and lead to a heart attack.

been shown time and again to lower the risk of heart attack in those who have angina.

Beta blockers can occasionally cause problems with blood sugar control in women with Type I (insulin-dependent) diabetes (see Diabetes, below), but with close monitoring these problems can usually be managed. Since diabetic women of all ages are at the highest risk for CAD, the benefit of these drugs outweighs the risk.

Older versions of beta blockers such as propranolol and timolol sometimes cause depression or fatigue as well as slow pulse, dizziness, diarrhea, cold or tingling fingers or toes, and dry mouth, eyes, or skin. Less often, people using these older beta blockers may develop insomnia, hallucinations, anxiety, confusion, or breathing difficulties (the drugs should be used with caution by people with asthma). But newer, more "cardioselective" drugs (atenolol, metoprolol) are less likely to cause these side effects.

Calcium-channel blockers. An alternative for women with typical angina or arterial spasm is a class of drugs called calcium-channel blockers (nifedipine, verapamil, diltiazem). Calcium-channel blockers keep the arteries from going into spasm by impeding the flow of calcium through the muscle cells lining the coronary arteries. Women with microvascular angina may need no treatment at all. If chest pain is troubling, however, calcium-channel blockers often relieve it.

Aspirin. Aspirin has become a mainstay in the prevention of angina caused by coronary artery disease. It acts in part by reducing the stickiness of platelets—blood components that play an important role in the formation of blockages within arteries (see illustration). A low dose of aspirin each day reduces the risk of future heart attacks in women with angina and CAD.

ACE inhibitors. Although this class of drugs (angiotensin converting enzyme inhibitors) is not used directly as a treatment for angina, studies have shown that they protect against future heart attacks in women with coronary artery disease. They are also effective in treating hypertension, another risk factor for heart attack.

Estrogen replacement therapy. The possible link between microvascular angina and falling estrogen levels has led to the suggestion of using estrogen as a therapy for this type of angina. At least one small study of women with microvascular angina showed that estrogen relieved chest pain. In women with coronary artery disease, there is evidence that estrogen replacement therapy after menopause slows the progression of their heart disease.

Surgery. If angina resulting from atherosclerosis does not respond to medications, procedures such as coronary angioplasty or coronary artery bypass surgery may be necessary (see Coronary Artery Disease), although some studies have indicated that such treatments may not be as effective in women as in men.

▸ How can angina be prevented?

Long-term treatment and prevention involves eliminating the risk factors that predispose some people to angina. For women who are overweight, this may mean losing excess pounds (which also decreases the risk of developing diabetes, another serious risk factor for CAD). For women who smoke, it means cutting out cigarettes. Controlling high blood pressure or elevated cholesterol should also be part of the plan.

Although exercise can trigger an angina attack, usually with medication and physical supervision a patient does not have to abandon it. A sedentary lifestyle may in itself increase the risk of heart disease. Although it makes sense for people with angina to stop exercising at the first sign of chest pain, there is good reason to adopt a moderate program of exercise under a clinician's supervision. Cardiac rehabilitation programs usually provide guidance in this.

Estrogen replacement therapy (see below) is becoming a mainstay in the heart disease prevention program of many women and should be considered by those entering menopause.

Arrhythmia

Abnormalities in the rhythm of the heart are called arrhythmias. They can range in severity from the incidental skipped beat to life-threatening emergencies. If palpitations or other kinds of heart irregularity are noted—and are not easily attributed to strenuous exercise, drinking too much coffee, or emotional upset—a physician should be consulted to rule out a possibly serious medical cause. The good news is that while some arrhythmias can be cause for worry, advances in treating them mean that the prognosis is good in most cases.

The heart's chemical-electrical system regulates the action of its chambers, allowing blood to be pumped efficiently to meet the body's needs. The signal starts in the "pacemaker" area of the heart, the sino-atrial node, or S-A node (see illustration). The S-A node sends out a regular electrical signal, about once a second, prompting other cells in the heart to contract and push blood into the ventricles. At another node, the atrio-ventricular or A-V node, the flow of blood is stopped for a moment, allowing the ventricles to fill with blood, to be pumped on and delivered to the lungs and the rest of the body.

Arrhythmias occur when the signal is interrupted somewhere along this path. Coronary artery disease can reduce the blood supply and lead to the "electrical death" associated with heart attacks. Arrhythmias can also occur when the heart tissue is stretched (as in Heart Failure; see below), when electrolytes such as potassium in the blood become imbalanced, and when stress or excitement raises the epinephrine levels in the blood. A number of substances (caffeine, alcohol, cocaine) can also cause arrhythmias.

▸ Types of arrhythmias

There are many types, but most fall into the following 6 patterns.

Premature contractions. A thump in the chest is caused by a premature signal arising somewhere in the heart. The chambers contract earlier than normal, breaking step with the regular heart-

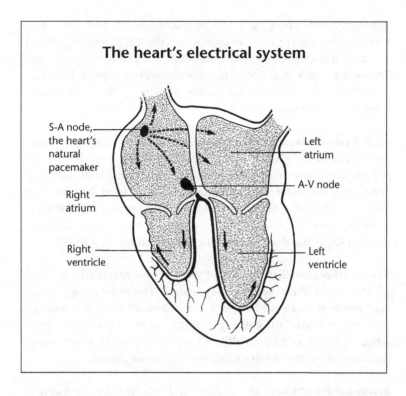

The heart's electrical system

S-A node,
the heart's
natural
pacemaker

Left
atrium

A-V node

Right
atrium

Right
ventricle

Left
ventricle

beat. Infrequent premature contractions are common and do not require treatment; they can be brought on by anxiety or simply by smoking or overindulgence of caffeine. They can also occur without any discernible triggering event.

Paroxysmal atrial tachycardia (PAT). Abnormal conduction pathways in the atria cause a fast, regular, often pounding heartbeat accompanied by a feeling of lightheadedness. Common in young, otherwise healthy adults, PAT usually can be treated with lifestyle modification (such as eliminating the use of caffeine, nicotine, and other stimulants and avoiding strenuous exertion) and if necessary with antiarrhythmic drugs.

Ventricular tachycardia (VT). Like PAT, ventricular tachycardia can be characterized by attacks of rapid heartbeat and dizziness, sometimes with chest pain. It can also be silent, and can cause fainting. The patient often describes "a feeling that something bad is going to happen." VT is far more serious than PAT, since it can degenerate into a fatal ventricular fibrillation (see below). This type of arrhythmia almost always occurs together with other serious heart disease. Immediate medical attention is essential.

Atrial fibrillation (AF). Random, chaotic electrical impulses in the atria cause the chambers of the heart to pump inefficiently. The pulse is rapid and irregular. This type of arrhythmia is usually seen in patients with heart disease, although it can occur in those with an overactive thyroid and in otherwise healthy people. If blood clots develop in the heart as a result of AF and break away to travel through the aorta, the consequence can sometimes be a stroke.

Ventricular fibrillation (VF). This pattern occurs when electrical activity in the ventricles becomes chaotic. The heart muscle tissue does not beat in a coordinated manner. Instead there is a series of localized twitching or writhing movements and no true pumping action. After a few minutes all heart activity ceases. VF is frequently the cause of sudden death in patients with heart disease.

Bradycardia. "Brady" means slow, and this term simply means a slow heart beat, strictly defined as a rate slower than 60 beats per minute (bpm). Problems do not usually occur until the heart rate falls below 40 bpm. Many healthy people, especially athletes, have heartbeats well below 60 bpm. But since a slow heart rate can signal inefficient heart action and possible oxygen deprivation to tissues and organs, a visit to the doctor can rule out bradycardia caused by a malfunctioning S-A node or a problem with the A-V node known as a heart block. Certain drugs can also cause bradycardia, particularly in the elderly.

‣ Who is likely to develop arrhythmia?
People with underlying heart disease—particularly coronary artery disease—are more likely to develop arrhythmias. Other factors associated with an increased risk are an enlarged heart for any reason, pregnancy, mitral valve prolapse (see Heart Valve Disorders) and an

overactive thyroid gland. Arrhythmias are also more likely—and can be fatal—in women with severe anorexia nervosa, an eating disorder in which people, usually young women, deliberately starve themselves.

▸ What are the symptoms?
An arrhythmia is often signaled by a racing or pounding heart, especially when the episode begins suddenly in the absence of exertion or emotional upset. The medical term for a racing heartbeat or a single skipped beat is palpitation. Arrhythmias are mostly experienced as palpitations, but because of the reduced supply of oxygen to the brain they can also be experienced as episodes of fatigue, faintness, or blackout.

▸ How is the condition evaluated?
Once an arrhythmia is suspected, the physician's initial goal is to determine the nature of the irregular heartbeat by ordering an electrocardiogram, or ECG. Because arrhythmias come and go and often elude detection during a visit to the doctor, a lightweight miniaturized electrocardiograph, the Holter monitor, may have to be worn on the belt for 24 hours. This device provides a record that can be analyzed by computer. Very complex rhythm problems may call for electrophysiological testing (in which tiny electrodes are threaded through the veins and planted directly in the heart). This procedure requires hospital admission and is performed by cardiologists with specialized training in this area.

▸ How is arrhythmia treated?
Most arrhythmias requiring a doctor's attention can be treated with drugs called antiarrhythmics, the most common ones being quinidine, digoxin, procainamide, and disopyramide. Propranolol (a beta blocker) and verapamil (a calcium-channel blocker) are frequently used as well. All of these drugs work by correcting the electrical imbalances that cause the irregular heartbeat.

Permanent pacemakers can correct the slow heartbeat caused by a heart block by overriding the heart's S-A node to initiate regular contractions of the ventricles. A pacemaker is about 3 inches square and is implanted under the skin, usually just below the collarbone.

It consists of a battery and one or two leads whose tips are positioned in the right side of the heart. There are various types of pacemakers, and some last up to 15 years before having to be replaced.

In the case of ventricular fibrillation, metal paddles are placed on the patient's chest to deliver a large dose of current that shocks the heart back into a regular rhythm. This procedure, which must happen within 3 minutes of the onset of fibrillation if the patient is to survive, is often performed by emergency room physicians or by paramedics in an ambulance or in a patient's home.

▸ How can arrhythmia be prevented?

The best prevention for some arrhythmia is to reduce one's risk factors for coronary artery disease. Since coffee, alcohol, and cigarettes, as well as extremely low-calorie diets, can cause some types of arrhythmias, lifestyle changes in these areas may also be in order.

Recent research suggests that while stress and strong emotions can contribute to an episode of arrhythmia, emotions alone probably do not have a direct cause-and-effect relationship to the incidence of life-threatening rhythm disturbances. Out of every 10 people seen for such an episode, the study suggested, 8 had not experienced any extraordinary emotion, positive or negative, in the 24 hours before their arrhythmia. When there was a link between emotion and arrhythmia, anger was a more likely trigger than fear or grief.

Far more likely to trigger an episode of arrhythmia was extreme fatigue. It seems likely that emotional distress, in conjunction with other factors such as fatigue, may make the heart more susceptible to a sudden spasm in an artery or to a spontaneous abnormality in the action of the heart. But emotions alone do not trigger the arrhythmia. This is comforting news for patients and their families after the diagnosis of heart disease and during recuperation from a heart-related illness. There is no need for family members to "walk on eggshells" or for patients to give up an active life with all its attendant emotions.

Coronary Artery Disease

Coronary artery disease is a form of heart disease caused by obstructions in the arteries that supply the heart with blood. Although CAD is the number-one killer of both men and women in this country, on average it tends to affect women about 10 or 15 years later in life.

This difference is thought to be due to the protective effect of the hormone estrogen in premenopausal women, which seems somehow to stall the progression of atherosclerosis—the process in which fat and cholesterol are deposited in the arteries (see illustration). There is some evidence that estrogen may have other protective effects as well, such as dilating the blood vessels and keeping them from going into spasm (which can cut off blood flow), as well as reducing the likelihood of dangerous blood clots.

Coronary artery disease is actually a continuum of atherosclerotic conditions, the most mild of which may involve no symptoms. As atherosclerosis progresses, however, scar tissue and other debris are deposited inside the muscular wall of the coronary arteries—the main arteries that supply the heart muscle with blood (see illustration). This can result in angina, a kind of chest pain that often follows exercise or emotional stress. When one or more coronary arteries are seriously narrowed, a heart attack (myocardial infarction) may result.

During a heart attack, cells in part of the heart cease functioning because they are so severely deprived of blood. Unless the blocked artery is opened promptly, this injury will be permanent and, depending on the extent of muscle death and its location, may be fatal. If the heart attack has been precipitated by a blood clot that has lodged in the narrowed artery, as is often the case, it is called coronary thrombosis.

▸ **Who is likely to develop coronary artery disease?**
Women do not have to worry about one of the major risk factors for coronary artery disease: maleness. The mere fact of being a man increases the odds of developing CAD by a factor of 3.5. Some of this female advantage may be attributable to differences in blood choles-

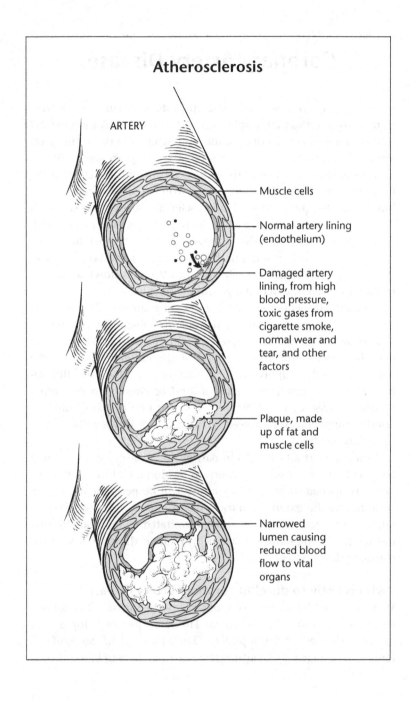

Atherosclerosis

ARTERY

Muscle cells

Normal artery lining (endothelium)

Damaged artery lining, from high blood pressure, toxic gases from cigarette smoke, normal wear and tear, and other factors

Plaque, made up of fat and muscle cells

Narrowed lumen causing reduced blood flow to vital organs

Coronary circulation and blockage

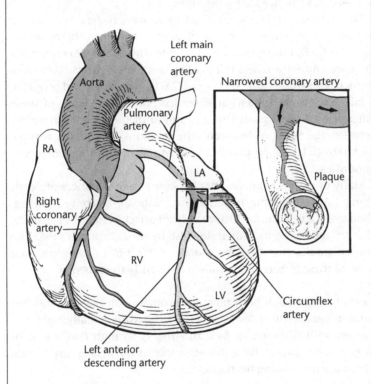

The right and left coronary arteries and their branches provide the blood supply to the heart muscle. When plaques develop within the vessels, the blood flow through them is diminished.
RA = right atrium
RV = right ventricle
LA = left atrium
LV = left ventricle

terol levels between men and premenopausal women. The fact that a woman's risk of developing CAD increases greatly after menopause—when blood cholesterol levels take on a more male pattern—lends credence to this possibility.

The biggest risk factor for CAD in women is age. The older a woman is, the greater are her chances of developing atherosclerosis and thus CAD. Ethnicity also plays a role. The rate of CAD is highest in African American men, followed by white men, African American women, and white women. Rates of CAD in Hispanics and people of Asian descent are somewhat lower for both sexes. Some of these differences may be related to anatomical or functional differences between the sexes or between ethnic groups, but others may be related to lack of appropriate referral and treatment for women and minorities.

Many of the same factors that increase a man's chances of developing CAD—including hypertension, diabetes, cigarette smoking, cholesterol levels, family history of heart attack before the age of 60, obesity, and a sedentary lifestyle—also increase a woman's risk. The limited studies that have been done so far, however, suggest that some of these factors affect women differently than men.

Diabetes. Although both men and women with diabetes mellitus are at increased risk of developing CAD, the risk is actually higher for women with diabetes. In fact, this risk is so high (twice that of women who do not have diabetes) that it outweighs any female advantage in avoiding heart disease.

Cholesterol. The significance of various blood cholesterol and lipid levels also varies between the sexes. In women, having low levels of HDL (high-density lipoprotein) cholesterol and high triglycerides may increase the odds of developing CAD, whereas in men high levels of LDL (low-density lipoprotein) cholesterol seem to be more problematic. High levels of triglycerides (a kind of fat molecule) appear to be a risk factor for coronary artery disease in women but not in men.

Sedentary lifestyle. Whether women are more sedentary than men—and thus at particularly high risk for CAD—remains questionable. Lack of exercise increases the risk of CAD in both sexes, and physical activity levels decrease with age, but it is not clear that women actually get less exercise than men. This is because questionnaires typically used to measure physical activity were developed primarily for men and may overlook the amount of energy that women expend doing housework, caring for children, gardening, and engaging in other nonsport activities.

Obesity. Although obesity is also considered to be a risk factor for CAD in men, this is only because men who are obese tend to have other risk factors for CAD at the same time (such as high blood pressure). In women the mere fact of being obese increases the chances of developing CAD, even in the absence of other factors. Women who have a relatively high waist-to-hip measurement ratio in particular appear to be at increased risk.

Risk factors unique to women. Women who have had their ovaries removed before natural menopause are at increased risk for developing coronary artery disease. Hysterectomy (the removal of the uterus) does not increase the risks, so long as at least one ovary is retained. Natural menopause, in and of itself, does not increase the risks of CAD either, but it does take away the protective effect of estrogen. Consequently, after menopause the risk of CAD goes up as women age. One might say that it is aging that causes CAD, not menopause; estrogen just delays the aging of the cardiovascular system until later in life.

As for the use of oral contraceptives, recent data indicate that there is no increased risk of CAD in women under 30 or in nonsmoking women over 30—unless these women have other cardiac risk factors. Earlier findings associating birth control pills with heart attacks were based on studies using pills with much higher doses of estrogen and progesterone than those commonly prescribed today.

The rate of CAD is 3 times higher for women in blue-collar occupations than for women in white-collar positions. The stress many women experience balancing roles as worker, wife, mother, housekeeper, and caretaker of elderly parents may also indirectly contribute to other risk factors such as smoking, hypertension, and obesity. Some studies have suggested that working women who have an

unsupportive supervisor, limited job mobility, or suppressed hostility appear to be at increased risk for developing CAD.

▸ What are the symptoms?

The symptoms of coronary artery disease range from none at all
to angina to heart attack to sudden cardiac death (the instantane-
ous cessation of heartbeat). Just which symptoms appear depends
on the degree of damage in the coronary arteries, as well as on the
person's sex.

For many men the first symptom of CAD is a heart attack, but
women are more likely to develop the chest pains of angina as their
first symptom. And when women do have heart attacks, they are
more likely than men to have pain, nausea, breathing difficulties,
and fatigue in addition to chest pain. Although men with CAD are
more likely than women to experience sudden cardiac death, CAD
still accounts for about one third of deaths from heart disease in
women. Two thirds of these sudden cardiac deaths among women
occur without any earlier symptoms of CAD.

▸ How is the condition evaluated?

The three methods most commonly used today to evaluate coronary artery disease are exercise stress testing, thallium scanning, and
coronary angiography.

Exercise stress test. This test, also called exercise electrocardiogra-
phy or exercise tolerance test (ETT), is used to evaluate the availability of blood to the heart during the stress of exercise. Electrodes
attached to wires are pasted onto the arms, legs, and chest, and the
heart's electrical activity is measured by a machine while the person
walks or jogs on a treadmill.

In most medical centers women with symptoms of heart disease
such as chest pain are much less likely than men with similar symptoms to receive a stress electrocardiogram, and when they are given
stress tests, their hearts seem to respond differently to exercise than
men's and give different readings. Too often women who show signs
of CAD on an exercise stress test turn out to have perfectly normal
arteries, while women who show no signs of CAD on the test turn
out to have blocked arteries. This high rate of false positives and
false negatives may be traced in part to the fact that, until quite

recently, exercise stress testing was developed and validated primarily on men. The fact that women are less likely to be able to do all the physical tasks required by the test may also help explain some of the false negatives.

Thallium scanning. Another kind of testing, called thallium scanning, is often done in conjunction with an exercise ECG or when a resting ECG is abnormal. It involves injecting a small amount of radioactive material into a vein and then using a scanner to detect emitted radiation. The amount of radiation emitted reflects the amount of blood that has reached various parts of the heart muscle.

Women undergo thallium scanning much less often than men, and their lower tolerance for exercise leads to a high number of false negatives in women who do have thallium stress testing. One solution for women unable to exercise is to use drugs called pharmacologic stressors, which dilate the blood vessels as though the women were actually exercising.

Stress tests are designed to stratify risk: they tell the clinician who is likely to have significant (and possibly dangerous) CAD. The results of the tests often indicate whether medicine or surgery should be the next step. If the stress tests are equivocal or ominous, catheterization will be used to assess the exact degree of blockage and from that one can decide whether to do angioplasty or coronary bypass surgery.

Coronary angiography. The most accurate tool to evaluate a woman suspected of having CAD is coronary angiography, also known as cardiac catheterization. In this procedure, a catheter (hollow tube) is guided into a coronary artery and then an opaque contrast agent is injected through it to make the blood visible on a moving x-ray image (see illustration). The result is a detailed picture of blood flow to the heart as well as a depiction of any blockages in the arteries. Before a patient undergoes any type of surgery for coronary artery disease, a coronary catheterization must be performed.

According to some studies, white women with abnormal ECGs, typical angina, and risk factors for CAD are much less likely than white men to be referred for this test—at least in some medical centers. African Americans of both sexes, but especially women, are

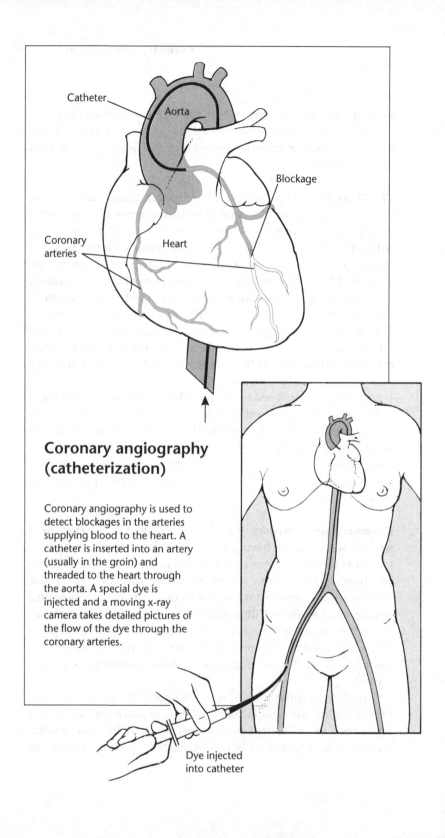

Catheter

Aorta

Blockage

Coronary
arteries

Heart

Coronary angiography
(catheterization)

Coronary angiography is used to
detect blockages in the arteries
supplying blood to the heart. A
catheter is inserted into an artery
(usually in the groin) and
threaded to the heart through
the aorta. A special dye is
injected and a moving x-ray
camera takes detailed pictures of
the flow of the dye through the
coronary arteries.

Dye injected
into catheter

even less likely to be offered cardiac angiography. It is unclear from the data whether the test is being done too often in white men, or not being done often enough in women and in African American men.

Even though the likelihood of serious CAD is lower in women than in men overall, if a woman has symptoms and risk factors, her physician should take an aggressive approach to her evaluation, including ordering stress tests and possibly catheterization when circumstances warrant it.

Echocardiography. Faced with all of these uncertainties in how to evaluate CAD in women, clinicians are beginning to consider alternative noninvasive tests that may be more appropriate. A type of ultrasound called exercise echocardiography seems to be particularly useful in detecting blockage in a single blood vessel—which is a common form of CAD in women. Echocardiography uses reflected sound waves from the heart to generate an image that corresponds to the direction and velocity of the blood flow. It can be used with exercise or in combination with pharmacologic stressors to simulate the effect of exercise.

‣ How is CAD treated?

Coronary artery disease can be treated with either medication or surgery, together with an attempt to control or eliminate risk factors such as high blood pressure or smoking. Just which approach is chosen depends on the patient's age, general health, and severity of heart-related symptoms.

Nitrates. Nitrates (nitroglycerin, Isordil, Ismo) are thought to increase blood flow to the heart by dilating coronary arteries. When used to treat an attack of angina (chest pain), a nitrate tablet is held under the tongue until it dissolves. Other forms can be swallowed for longer protection against chest pain. Nitrate ointments can also be rubbed directly into the chest or arm, or, for slower release, applied as a patch soaked with nitrate and covered with adhesive plastic. Over time, nitrate patches lose their effectiveness. The few studies that have been done on women with angina indicate that nitrates may not be as effective in reducing either the frequency or intensity of symptoms as in men.

ACE inhibitors. This class of drugs has been shown to have a positive effect on heart function and a protective effect against future heart attacks in women with CAD. Angiotensin converting enzyme inhibitors also lower blood pressure, with relatively few side effects.

Beta blockers. These drugs work by lowering the heart's demand for blood. Normally the heartbeat is stimulated by chemical messengers sent through the nerves to sites in the heart called beta adrenergic receptors. In a person with CAD, blocked coronary arteries diminish blood supply to the heart, and the nerves respond by sending out plenty of this chemical messenger. The heart beats faster and requires a faster blood flow, but the blocked arteries still cannot respond. The result is the pain of angina.

Beta-blocking drugs relieve this pain by slipping into the sites that would otherwise be filled by the chemical messengers, thus keeping the heart from beating faster and thereby allowing more time for the coronary arteries to fill.

Beta blockers, however, also slip into beta receptors in other parts of the body, sometimes producing uncomfortable side effects such as breathing difficulties, depression, and fatigue. Propranolol (Inderal), an older beta blocker, may cause such unwanted effects. Some of the side effects can be avoided with the newer, more expensive beta blockers (called cardioselective beta blockers) which enter only beta receptors in the heart. Atenolol (Tenormin) is a widely used cardioselective beta blocker.

Calcium-channel blockers. These medications keep the arteries from going into spasm and temporarily restricting the flow of blood. Coronary artery spasms are a particularly common cause of chest pain in women. They seem to be switched on by the mineral calcium, which is dissolved in the blood and body fluids and enters channels that begin outside the wall of the blood vessels. Calcium-channel blockers fill these channels, thus preventing the entrance of calcium into the vessel and any resulting spasm (see Angina Pectoris, above).

Various calcium-channel blockers are available, including verapamil (Calan), diltiazem (Cardizem), and nifedipine (Procardia),

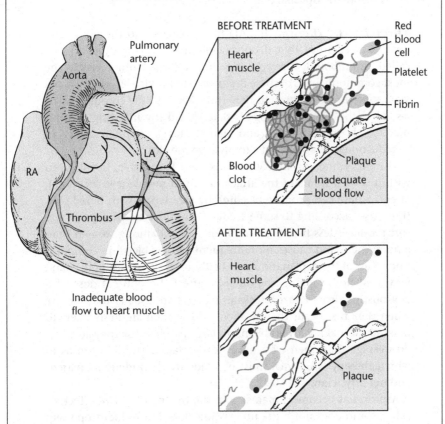

Clot busters

BEFORE TREATMENT

Pulmonary artery

Aorta

Heart muscle

Red blood cell

Platelet

Fibrin

LA

RA

Blood clot

Plaque

Thrombus

Inadequate blood flow

AFTER TREATMENT

Heart muscle

Inadequate blood flow to heart muscle

Plaque

When a blood clot (thrombus) in a coronary artery disrupts the flow of blood to part of the heart muscle, lack of oxygen (ischemia) can cause permanent damage unless the clot is dissolved promptly. Thrombolytic drugs break up the blockage, which consists of long strands of fibrin (a protein), red blood cells, and platelets.

each of which varies somewhat in its efficacy against different aspects of CAD. Often it is necessary to try more than one of these drugs before the optimal one is found.

Thrombolytic therapy. If CAD has progressed to the point of a heart attack, drugs that dissolve clots may be employed. This is called thrombolytic therapy (see illustration). Until recently the most commonly used of these drugs was streptokinase, administered via a tube threaded through the arm or leg into the coronary arteries. After the site of blockage is determined (by inserting contrast material through the tube and taking x-rays), streptokinase is injected through the same tube to dissolve the clot.

The procedure can be complicated and is invasive, but if given within several hours of the attack, for most people it is successful. Streptokinase can produce bleeding by interfering with blood clotting. Also, according to some studies, thrombolytic therapy of any sort produces less benefit in terms of survival among women than among men, and causes more frequent serious bleeding complications. Part of the explanation may be that we still do not understand very well how weight, age, and sex affect the optimal dose of a clot-busting drug. Heart attacks in women are usually more severe when they first occur than in men, and women are more likely to have additional health problems, in large part because they are older on average than men who have heart attacks. The decision as to which therapy is optimal must be made by the individual patient and her physician.

Aspirin has become a mainstay in the treatment of CAD. Technically aspirin does not break up existing clots, but it does stop them from increasing in size. For this reason aspirin is given immediately to any person suspected of having a heart attack in progress. It is also given to people with known CAD or more than two risk factors for heart disease, to reduce the chances of future heart attacks and stroke.

Balloon angioplasty. In this surgical procedure the physician inserts a thin catheter with a balloon at the end into the artery and pushes it into the blocked area. As the balloon is expanded, it pushes the obstruction aside and opens up a passage for blood flow. Con-

Conventional balloon angioplasty

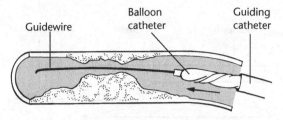

Guidewire   Balloon catheter   Guiding catheter

A guiding catheter is positioned in the opening of the coronary artery and a thin, flexible guidewire is pushed down the vessel and through the narrowed artery. The balloon catheter is then advanced over this guidewire.

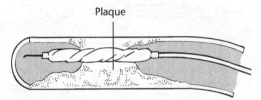

Plaque

The balloon catheter is positioned next to the atherosclerotic plaque.

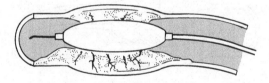

The balloon is inflated, stretching and cracking the plaque.

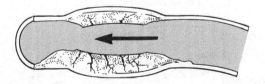

When the balloon is withdrawn, blood flow is reestablished through the widened vessel.

Coronary stent

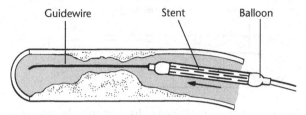

Guidewire   Stent   Balloon

A special catheter with a deflated balloon and a stent at the tip is used to place a stent within a narrowed vessel.

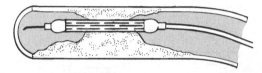

The catheter is positioned so that the stent is within the narrowed region of the coronary artery.

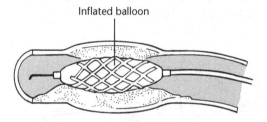

Inflated balloon

The balloon is then inflated, causing the stent to expand and stretch the coronary artery.

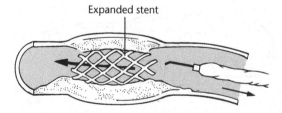

Expanded stent

The balloon catheter is then withdrawn, leaving the stent behind to keep the vessel open.

Coronary atherectomy

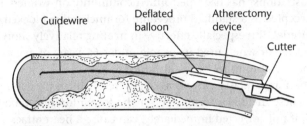

Guidewire Deflated balloon Atherectomy device Cutter

A special device with a deflated balloon on one side and an opening on the other is pushed over a wire down the coronary artery to the narrowing.

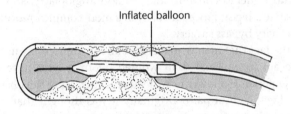

Inflated balloon

When the balloon is inflated, part of the plaque is "squeezed" into the opening of the device.

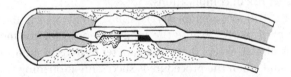

As the cutting blade is rotated, pieces of plaque are shaved off into the device.

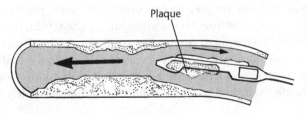

Plaque

The catheter is withdrawn, leaving a larger opening for blood flow.

ventional balloon angioplasty (along with its more recent relatives; see illustrations) has been performed commonly on women and is now accepted as a standard procedure for unclogging blocked coronary arteries. It is especially effective in treating relatively short areas of blockage or when used in people under 65 years of age or who have had symptoms for only a short time.

Balloon angioplasty can occasionally result in serious complications. These include a torn artery or the formation of a blood clot which, if not corrected immediately, can cause a heart attack rather than prevent one. These complications are very rare when the procedure is performed by an experienced cardiologist. Of more concern is the fact that arteries will narrow again within a year in 1 out of 3 patients who undergo conventional balloon angioplasty, and that may necessitate a repeat procedure or even a more complex procedure such as coronary bypass surgery.

Despite the fact that men who receive balloon angioplasty usually have more advanced CAD than women, women who have this procedure experience a lower rate of success at clearing the obstruction and relieving chest pain. Originally it was thought that these differences might be due to the smaller size of women's arteries, so cardiologists tried using a smaller balloon. This modification has made very little difference. Now cardiologists believe that women's relatively greater age and coexisting health problems account for their higher risk of complications.

Even so, balloon angioplasty is still a good option for many women, particularly because the long-term outcome for men and women is similar, except that chest pain tends to recur more often in women. And when the procedure is successful at opening women's arteries, the blood vessels are less likely than men's to become blocked again.

Coronary bypass surgery. In this operation a short piece of vein from the thigh or the internal mammary artery (IMA) from the chest is grafted onto a narrowed coronary artery to reroute blood around a blockage (see illustration). There is abundant evidence that this surgery is effective in relieving anginal pain that has not responded to medications, as well as for CAD in 3 arteries or in the left main

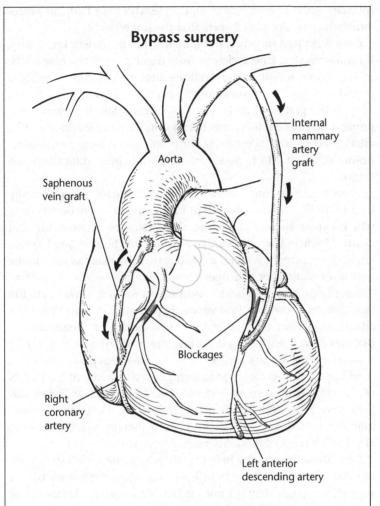

Bypass surgery

Internal
mammary
artery
graft

Aorta

Saphenous
vein graft

Blockages

Right
coronary
artery

Left anterior
descending artery

Two types of grafts can be used for bypassing obstructed coronary arteries. A portion of the saphenous vein (taken from the leg) can be used to connect the aorta to the right coronary artery just beyond the blockage. The internal mammary artery, freed from its usual position in the chest wall, can be connected to the left anterior descending artery at a point past the obstruction. Arrows show the new direction of blood flow.

coronary artery. About half of all people who have had this procedure remain free of pain 5 years after the surgery.

Even so, bypass surgery is not something to be undertaken lightly. It cannot prevent atherosclerosis from developing in the new grafts. In fact, some recent studies indicate that as many as 4 out of 5 people who have had bypass surgery develop life-threatening blockages in the graft within 10 years of surgery. The IMA seems less prone to subsequent blockages than a vein from the thigh; since this artery is being used increasingly, the problem may become less significant (although IMA bypasses are technically more difficult to perform).

There is still no consensus about whether bypass surgery actually lengthens life expectancy—except in the case of severe obstruction, where bypass surgery can mean the difference between life and death. Although both sexes are equally likely to be alive 5 to 10 years after bypass surgery, women are about twice as likely as men to die during or soon after the operation. This may be due in part to differences in body and blood vessel size in women, as well as to the fact that many women undergoing bypass surgery are older, have advanced disease, or have other serious health problems such as diabetes or congestive heart failure. More often than not, too, a woman having bypass surgery is in an emergency situation, and mortality rates therefore tend to be higher. Also, many of the studies of mortality in women were done when techniques of bypass surgery were less advanced than they are today. Using the internal mammary artery and routine antiplatelet therapy to prevent blood clotting has reduced mortality rates in both sexes.

All of these factors may help explain why women with symptoms of CAD may be less likely than men to be offered coronary bypass surgery, although they do not explain why African Americans of both sexes are less likely to undergo coronary artery bypass procedures for CAD than are whites. Yet, given the high cost of bypass surgery—not to mention the relatively high risk of complications and the risk of death from these complications (which vary from doctor to doctor and from hospital to hospital)—not having this surgery or any other surgery is not necessarily a bad thing. The consensus is that women with mild or moderate angina run no particular risk in delaying surgical procedures for CAD until they have first tried relieving their symptoms with drugs, diet, and exercise.

> **How can coronary artery disease be prevented?**

Coronary artery disease is the product of a number of variables, some of which (such as family history) cannot be controlled. It is nonetheless possible to lower the risk of CAD by changing certain habits that may precipitate risk factors. Giving up cigarettes, for example (or, better yet, never starting to smoke them), cuts the risk of mortality from CAD in half. More than 60 percent of heart attacks in women under the age of 50 can be attributed to cigarette smoking, and women who stop smoking after a heart attack have a longer life expectancy than women who continue to smoke.

Evidence is less clear on whether modifying other behaviors can lower risk, but there is some evidence that women who have had a heart attack can increase their chances of survival by controlling hypertension—even mild hypertension. As for improving blood fat and cholesterol levels, the benefits in women are not as clear as in men, although recent studies have suggested that there is some benefit in raising the relative proportion of high-density lipoprotein (HDL) to low-density lipoprotein (LDL) cholesterol and lowering triglycerides (see High Cholesterol). Usually clinicians advise women to increase exercise and eat a relatively low-fat diet, and, if necessary, to use medications to control extremely high blood cholesterol or lipid levels.

Compared with nondrinkers, women over 50 who consume 1 to 20 drinks a week appear to have a somewhat lower risk of heart disease, probably because alcohol seems to elevate levels of HDL cholesterol. The same effect appears to occur in men as well. This potential benefit has to be weighed against the well-known risks of alcohol consumption in women, which include alcohol dependence and liver damage (see Alcohol Use).

Although controversy continues, there is growing evidence that weight loss is an effective strategy against CAD. The link between obesity and CAD in women has been well established. But even a weight gain of 10 to 20 pounds in a middle-aged woman increases her future risk of coronary disease, according to some recent studies. Women who are overweight and have other risk factors for CAD should work with a clinician to find a safe and effective means of weight control. Exercise is usually an essential part of any weight-loss program, and seems to have other effects that are beneficial to the heart.

Women (as well as men) who have Type I (insulin-dependent) diabetes may be able to decrease their risk of heart disease by controlling their blood sugar level and using intensive insulin therapy. Whether this "tight control" is equally effective in people with Type II diabetes requires further investigation (see Diabetes).

New evidence suggests that daily use of small dosages of aspirin (1 regular strength or baby aspirin per day) in women aged 34 to 59 can reduce the chances of having a heart attack. After a heart attack many clinicians recommend using either aspirin or beta blockers to reduce the risk of a second heart attack. This therapy, widely prescribed for men, should be promoted for women as well.

Finally, women who already have CAD or who are at high risk for developing CAD should seriously consider estrogen replacement therapy (see below) after menopause. Although there are risks associated with this therapy, a high risk of CAD frequently overrides most of them.

Heart Failure

Heart failure (technically known as congestive heart failure) occurs when the heart fails to pump blood adequately, causing blood to back up in the veins that return it to the heart. As a result, tissues throughout the body are deprived of the oxygen which is normally transported by the blood. Backed-up blood causes fluid to collect in various parts of the body such as the lungs, lower legs, ankles, and liver.

Congestive heart failure can result from a variety of underlying problems, including mechanical problems of the heart valves, previous heart attacks, heart rhythm disturbances, damaged heart muscle, or long-standing high blood pressure. In women it is less likely to be associated with coronary artery disease than in men. Instead, it tends to involve problems with different parts of the pumping mechanism.

There are two phases to the pumping action of the heart: the "squeeze" (systole), when the heart muscle contracts and pumps blood through the arteries; and the "relaxation" (diastole), when the muscle relaxes and the heart fills with blood, ready to begin a new pumping cycle. The type of congestive heart failure caused by coronary artery disease (the type most common in men) occurs because damaged heart muscle loses its ability to "squeeze." In women, problems with the relaxation phase are more common. The heart muscle becomes stiffer or thickened and does not allow the heart to fill with blood. The most common cause is long-standing high blood pressure; the heart muscle enlarges and stiffens because it is forced to pump against high pressure in the arteries.

▸ Who is likely to develop congestive heart failure?

In both sexes, hypertension greatly increases the risk of developing congestive heart failure. Women with diabetes are also at particularly high risk because they are more prone to coronary artery disease, which causes scarring of heart muscle and loss of "squeeze." Congestive heart failure occurs more frequently in men than in women and strikes women at a later age, but women who develop it are much more likely to die from the disease.

▶ What are the symptoms?

The main symptoms of congestive heart failure are breathlessness, fatigue, weakness, and swelling (edema). Which of these symptoms occurs depends on which part of the heart is failing. If the pumping from the left side of the heart is inefficient, blood will back up into the lungs, leading them to become congested with fluid. The result is a condition called pulmonary edema, which is generally characterized by breathlessness. Often people with mild congestive heart failure become short of breath mainly with exertion. In later stages breathlessness is present even when the person is lying down or sitting.

If the right side of the heart is failing, backed-up blood congests the liver and the legs, resulting in swelling in the lower legs and ankles and liver malfunction. If blood flow to the kidneys is reduced, excess fluids will accumulate in tissues throughout the body, leading to more generalized edema. Swelling throughout the body, as well as breathlessness, will also occur if both sides of the heart are failing, which is often the case. In addition, inadequate blood flow to muscles leads to fatigue and weakness.

▶ How is the condition evaluated?

A clinician who suspects congestive heart failure will listen to the heart and lungs with a stethoscope and then conduct a number of tests of heart structure and function. These tests may include an electrocardiogram (ECG) to check for abnormalities in the heart's rate or rhythm and an echocardiogram to examine the heart's pumping action, as well as a chest x-ray. Various blood and urine tests will be done to evaluate kidney function.

▶ How is congestive heart failure treated?

There is no specific cure for most cases of congestive heart failure, but various steps can be taken to help people with this condition achieve a relatively normal life. Traditionally treatment has consisted of a combination of rest (to take some of the strain off the heart and other organs), salt-restricted diet (to reduce swelling), certain heart medications (such as digoxin) to increase the heart's pumping capacity, and other drugs (such as ACE inhibitors) to reduce the resistance to blood flow. In some cases surgery to repair or replace damaged heart muscle or valves is necessary. For the most severe cases heart transplantation is sometimes considered.

It now appears that some of the drugs commonly prescribed for congestive heart failure—including diuretics (which increase the output of salt and water by the kidneys, thereby decreasing the volume of blood and lowering blood pressure), digitalis (which increases the force of the heart's pumping action), and vasodilators (which widen the arteries and decrease resistance)—may not work for some women whose congestive heart failure is caused by the inability of the heart to fill adequately with blood. Other drugs, particularly beta blockers and calcium-channel blockers, may be used to treat this kind of congestive heart failure.

The outlook for people with congestive heart failure varies depending on the underlying condition. When an abnormal heart rhythm is the cause and can be treated, heart failure is unlikely to recur. Heart failure caused by longstanding high blood pressure or by minor damage to the heart from a heart attack can often be successfully treated with medication. When the heart muscle has been extensively damaged by a single large heart attack or multiple small attacks, the outlook is less encouraging; the patient's activity is likely to be drastically limited. Finally, global damage of the entire heart muscle from an infection, often caused by a virus, has the worst outlook: this condition, which can occur in relatively young people, may be successfully treated only with a heart transplant.

Heart Valve Disorders

▸Aortic Stenosis

In aortic stenosis the valve that separates the heart from the aorta—the main artery leaving the heart—narrows. As a result, the heart has to pump harder to keep the blood flowing through the valve, and the left ventricle (lower chamber) of the heart eventually becomes thickened and enlarged from its overexertion.

One of several forms of valvular heart disease, aortic stenosis is usually caused either by a congenital abnormality in the aortic valve or by age-related degeneration of the valve. This degeneration involves scarring and the build-up of calcium on the three flaps, or leaflets, of fibrous tissue that normally open and close the aortic valve (see illustration). This calcification, which restricts the size of the opening, tends to occur at an earlier age in women than in men.

▸Who is likely to develop aortic stenosis?

For reasons still unknown, as women age their valves calcify more quickly than men's. Thus, for the first 70 years of life, men are more likely than women to have aortic stenosis, but after the age of 70 aortic stenosis is more common in women. In either sex, symptoms are unlikely to appear before middle age. Occasionally, aortic valve problems (but not necessarily aortic stenosis per se) may occur in women who have had rheumatic heart disease—scarring of the heart valves following infection. This is particularly true in women who have immigrated to the United States from Southeast Asia, South America, or Central America, regions of the world where rheumatic fever, a rare complication of strep infections, is more prevalent.

▸What are the symptoms?

Because a narrowed aortic valve makes it difficult for the heart to pump blood through the valve and out to the body, various vital organs—not the least of which are the brain and the heart itself—become deprived of oxygen. The symptoms of aortic stenosis

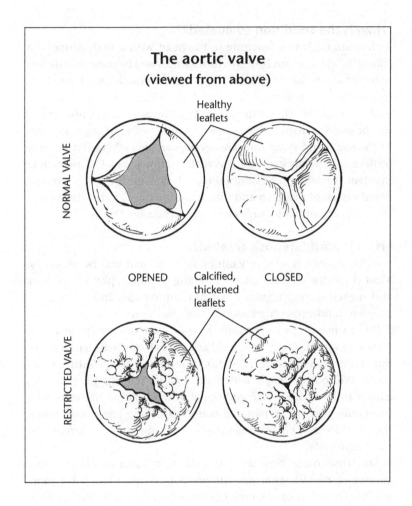

The aortic valve
(viewed from above)

Healthy leaflets

NORMAL VALVE

OPENED   Calcified, thickened leaflets   CLOSED

RESTRICTED VALVE

reflect this deprivation. For example, when the heart is deprived of blood, chest pain (angina) may result. When the brain is not getting enough oxygen, dizziness or fainting may result. Breathlessness is another common symptom—the body's reaction to its sense that not enough oxygen is reaching life-sustaining organs.

All of these symptoms tend to be most obvious during exercise, when oxygen demands are the highest, but as the condition worsens they may occur even during rest.

▸ How is the condition evaluated?

A clinician begins by listening to the heart with a stethoscope. If a characteristic murmur is heard, further tests will be done to differentiate aortic stenosis from several less serious conditions. These tests may include a chest x-ray to check for calcification on the valve as well as the overall size of the heart. An echocardiogram (ultrasound) will be done to inspect the narrowness of the valve. If aortic stenosis seems likely and symptoms are severe, cardiac catheterization may be necessary to measure how severe the narrowing is. This procedure involves threading a flexible tube (catheter) from the leg into the blood vessels of the heart and then passing a dye through the tube to show the extent of blockage (see Coronary Artery Disease).

▸ How is aortic stenosis treated?

If aortic stenosis is relatively minor, no treatment may be necessary. Most clinicians do recommend avoiding strenuous physical activity and suggest having regular physical examinations and echocardiograms to follow the progression of the condition.

If the valve is obstructed more significantly, or if symptoms have begun to appear, there are medications that can help temporarily. But surgery to replace or reconstruct the valve is the definitive treatment. Without it, people with serious aortic stenosis generally can expect to live only 2 or 3 additional years. Dilating the valve in a procedure using an expanding balloon (balloon angioplasty) does not seem to be as effective as valve surgery in ensuring a longer and more active life.

Abnormal blood flow around a diseased valve allows any tiny clumps of bacteria that may be present to infect the valve more readily. The result can be endocarditis—infection and inflammation of the membrane that covers the interior of the heart. To prevent this, people with aortic stenosis should use antibiotics before dental and certain surgical procedures, and should make sure their dentist is aware of their condition.

▸ Aortic regurgitation.

In this condition, the three leaflets that make up the aortic valve do not create a tight seal (see illustration). Consequently, blood leaks

Normal aortic valve

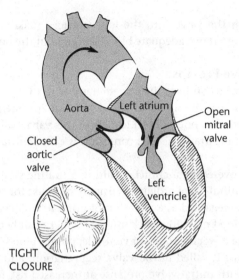

Between heartbeats, the left ventricle fills with blood that enters from the left atrium through the mitral valve. Normally, the three leaflets of the aortic valve close tightly and prevent blood in the aorta from leaking back into the heart.

Aortic regurgitation

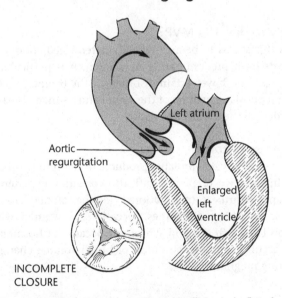

In people with aortic regurgitation or insufficiency, leaflets do not achieve a tight seal. Blood leaks (regurgitates) back through the valve into the left ventricle, increasing its work and eventually enlarging the heart.

back through the valve into the left ventricle, making it have to pump harder to move adequate blood throughout the body.

▸ Mitral Valve Prolapse

The mitral valve connects the upper chamber to the lower chamber on the left side of the heart. In about 1 out of 20 Americans, most frequently women, one or both leaflets of this valve balloon out, or prolapse (see illustration). This condition is called mitral valve prolapse (MVP).

Often discovered by a clinician during a routine stethoscope examination, mitral valve prolapse is usually no cause for concern and in fact can be regarded as a variation of normal. On occasion, however, some blood may flow back into the upper chamber, or atrium, whenever the lower chamber, or ventricle, pumps blood in the other direction. This is called mitral valve regurgitation, and it seems to put people with mitral valve prolapse at increased risk for infective endocarditis, an infection of the membrane that covers the interior of the heart. People with mitral valve prolapse are also at slightly higher risk for stroke. An association between mitral valve prolapse and panic disorder, though once suspected, has never been confirmed.

▸ Who is likely to develop MVP?

In some cases this seems to be a genetically determined condition which manifests itself predominantly in women. It is particularly common in those who have certain disorders of the thoracic skeleton, including scoliosis (curvature of the spine) and a sunken breastbone, or disorders of the connective tissue.

▸ What are the symptoms?

Most of the time mitral valve prolapse produces no symptoms whatsoever. Sometimes, however, people with this condition experience chest pain, rapid heartbeat (palpitations), fatigue, anxiety, lightheadedness, or breathing difficulties. Occasionally women with mitral valve prolapse will develop symptoms because of hormonal changes that occur during menstruation or blood volume changes that occur during pregnancy.

Flow to brain and body

Left
atrium

Aorta

Right
atrium

Flow from lungs

Mitral
valve

Left
ventricle

Right
ventricle

Normal mitral valve

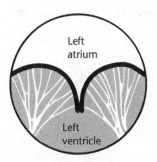

Left
atrium

Left
ventricle

Normally, the mitral valve closes tightly, and blood that has been pumped into the left ventricle does not reenter the left atrium.

Prolapsed mitral valve

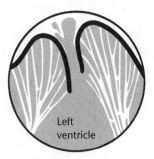

Left
ventricle

When the mitral valve does not make a tight seal, blood may reenter the left atrium—a condition called mitral valve regurgitation.

▸ How is the condition evaluated?

A characteristic click-murmur sound heard through a stethoscope often signals mitral valve prolapse to a clinician. The clicks occur because of the prolapse itself, and if blood flows back into the atrium, a murmur can be detected shortly thereafter. To confirm the diagnosis an echocardiogram may be done in a hospital's cardiac ultrasound department. This noninvasive and painless procedure transforms reflected sound waves into a continuous screen image of the heart tissues.

▸ How is mitral valve prolapse treated?

Most people with mitral valve prolapse require no treatment. In some individuals, however, a clinician may recommend taking antibiotics before dental work or surgery to reduce the risk of developing endocarditis from a bacterial infection.

If chest pain caused by palpitations is troublesome, these symptoms are usually treated with beta blockers (such as atenolol or propanolol). These drugs should be used with caution by people with asthma as they can occasionally worsen symptoms.

Other Associated Conditions

Diabetes

Diabetes mellitus is a group of disorders characterized by high levels of glucose (sugar) in the blood. All of them result from problems with insulin, a hormone that removes glucose from the blood and causes it to be stored in body cells. Type I and Type II diabetes are the most common forms, but up to 3 percent of women who did not previously have (or know they had) diabetes may develop it during pregnancy (a condition called gestational diabetes).

In Type I diabetes (also called juvenile diabetes) the pancreas—a long, soft, irregularly shaped gland located behind the stomach—does not produce enough insulin. Most people with Type I diabetes require regular injections of insulin for life. Although boys and girls run an equal risk of developing Type I until about age 12, around the time of puberty the incidence in females begins to decrease in comparison to that in males. Up to age 30 approximately 25 percent more men than women develop Type I, but later on the risk is about the same for men and women.

Most people who develop diabetes as adults have Type II, a form in which the body requires greater than normal amounts of insulin to maintain normal blood glucose levels, probably because cells throughout the body do not respond appropriately to insulin (see illustration). Type II (formerly called adult-onset diabetes) typically begins after the age of 40, often in people who are overweight or obese, and in those with a family history of diabetes. Whether men or women get Type II diabetes more often is still unsettled.

Gestational diabetes is a unique form of the disorder which occurs in pregnancy, probably as a result of hormones made by the placenta which alter the way insulin works. Although glucose levels usually return to normal after the baby is born, women who have gestational diabetes and required insulin during pregnancy do run a higher than average risk of developing Type II diabetes later in life.

How insulin works

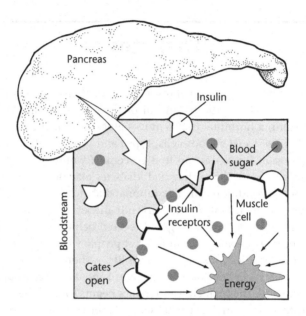

The pancreas secretes insulin into the bloodstream in response to a high level of blood sugar. The insulin molecules then bind to special insulin receptors on the surface of cells in muscles and other organs. The receptors signal the cell to allow sugar to enter, so that it can be available as a source of energy.

In people who are resistant to insulin, sugar has difficulty entering the cell even though insulin binds to the receptors.

Gestational diabetes most often occurs in pregnant women who are over the age of 30, who are obese, who have previously given birth to a very large (over 9 pounds) or stillborn baby, or who have a family history of diabetes.

▸ Who is at risk?

Compared with men of the same age, nondiabetic women seem to have a degree of protection from diseases of the heart and blood vessels until they reach menopause. Women with diabetes seem to lose this relative protection and at all ages are at increased risk of developing or dying from coronary artery disease, heart failure (inefficient pumping of the entire heart), strokes, and peripheral vascular disease. Cigarette smoking, hypertension, and obesity all magnify these risks.

In some cases women with diabetes are at higher risk than men with diabetes of the same age. The risk of dying from heart disease, for example, is higher for women than for men, though both men and women with the disease have a higher risk of dying from these problems than do people in the general population. This is partly because their blood vessels are often extensively damaged and partly because their heart attacks may involve unusual symptoms that make them harder to detect.

Certain operations commonly performed on patients with heart disease may be especially risky for women with diabetes. For example, some (but not all) studies suggest that coronary bypass surgery may be less effective and riskier in women with diabetes than in nondiabetic women. If this turns out to be true, it may have something to do with the nature of the fatty deposits in the arteries of women with diabetes. Whether diabetic women develop more complications from coronary angioplasty (balloon surgery) than do nondiabetic women or diabetic men is not known.

▸ How is diabetes treated?

Recent research has conclusively shown that normalizing blood glucose levels in Type I diabetics helps prevent coronary artery disease. Many doctors believe that this holds true for Type II diabetics as well.

The strategy for controlling blood glucose for Type I diabetics is to watch diet, maintain a regular exercise program, and adjust insulin dosages carefully according to frequent blood glucose measurements. A woman can check her own glucose level several times a day at home with a simple device called a glucometer. The patient takes a small lancet, pricks the end of a finger lightly, and puts a drop of blood on a strip of paper, which is placed into a small machine. After a minute the reading appears.

For the majority of women with Type II diabetes, weight control is an especially important strategy for controlling blood glucose. For women who are overweight, a return to normal body weight can bring blood glucose to normal levels. Maintaining a healthy body weight may even help prevent Type II diabetes from developing. If blood glucose cannot be controlled by attention to weight (through exercise and diet), insulin therapy or oral medications—for example, oral hypoglycemics and newer medications such as metformin (Glucophage)and troglitazone (Rezulin)—are the next step. In addition, health practices that make sense for everybody—such as getting regular exercise and avoiding cigarettes—are particularly important for people with diabetes.

Estrogen replacement therapy (ERT) in postmenopausal women, especially those with diabetes, may help reduce the risk of some forms of cardiovascular disease. Preliminary evidence suggests that ERT may slightly improve glucose control in women with diabetes, and it has beneficial effects on cholesterol levels, which, when elevated in diabetics, compound the risk of heart disease. The risks of ERT do not appear to be any higher for women with diabetes than for other women.

High Blood Pressure

Consistently high blood pressure—hypertension—is a common problem in the United States and is considered a major cause of heart disease and stroke. At least 1 in 5 American adults is thought to have high blood pressure. Although the disease is more common in men than in women overall, the numbers balance out with age because women tend to live longer.

Hypertension is not a unitary condition with a single cause but seems to result from a combination of environmental influences in people who are genetically susceptible. There are two basic forms: primary and secondary. Primary hypertension (sometimes called essential hypertension), which accounts for the vast majority of cases, arises on its own without any underlying disease or disorder. In contrast, secondary (or organic) hypertension results from some preexisting condition.

Blood pressure is the amount of pressure exerted by the blood against the arterial walls. It is measured twice: during a contraction of the heart muscle (systolic blood pressure) and during the longer periods of rest between contractions (diastolic blood pressure). Thus, a blood pressure measurement always consists of two numbers, such as 120/80 (read as "120 over 80"). In this case, 120 stands for the systolic pressure, while 80 stands for the diastolic pressure. The systolic pressure is always higher than the diastolic pressure.

A clinician measures blood pressure by using a sphygmomanometer or similar device. The sphygmomanometer consists of a rubber cuff that wraps around the arm just above the crook of the elbow and is connected to a calibrated tube filled with mercury. By pumping the cuff with air so that it squeezes the arm and then listening for pulse sounds with a stethoscope, the clinician gets a numerical reading that corresponds to the height of a column of mercury supported by the blood pressure. Thus, a systolic reading of 120 means that the blood pressure during the contraction of the heart supported a column of mercury 120 millimeters high.

Blood pressure is affected by many factors, some of which are longstanding—such as the pumping power of the heart or the resistance (elasticity and smoothness) of the arteries. But many more transient factors can also account for blood pressure changes: time of day, medications, or current level of emotional stress (including the stress of having one's blood pressure measured in the doctor's office!). Only a consistently high reading—measured in at least two different settings by competent clinicians with accurate equipment—is enough to justify a diagnosis of hypertension. The diagnosis of hypertension is not something to be made lightly, since it may result in a lifetime of medication.

There is disagreement within the medical community about just how high blood pressure has to be before it is considered hypertension. Different standards of interpretation are a major reason why estimates of the prevalence of high blood pressure often vary. The World Health Organization considers 160/95 to be the upper limit of the normal range, whereas the U.S. government's Joint National Committee on Detection, Evaluation, and Treatment of High Blood Pressure considers blood pressure at or over 160/90 to be a problem. Many insurance companies start raising their premiums for people with much lower levels, while American physicians routinely recommend that anyone with a diastolic blood pressure of 90 or more take steps to lower it, either with immediate lifestyle changes or with medication (or both).

Whether the same blood pressure should be considered dangerous in people of different age, sex, or ethnicity also remains the subject of debate. It is well known that various demographic factors have a major bearing on the consequences of hypertension. For example, serious complications are much more likely to develop in African Americans than in whites with the same degree of hypertension. Similarly, complications are much more likely to develop in men than in women with identical levels of hypertension.

▸ Who is likely to develop high blood pressure?

In the population at large, men are more likely than women to develop hypertension, and African Americans are more likely to develop it than whites. African American women over the age of 40 are twice as likely to have hypertension as white women of the same age. There seems to be a higher than average rate of hypertension among Filipinos and lower than average rates in people of Chinese or Hispanic descent. Because the prevalence of hypertension tends to increase with age, however, these general statements can be misleading. Although blood pressure in young white women tends to be lower than blood pressure in young white men, for example, white women aged 60 to 74 are just as likely as white men the same age to have hypertension. For African American women the statistics are grimmer: they are just as likely to have hypertension as African American men their age by the time they reach 45.

Excess sodium in the diet and inadequate potassium and calcium have all been linked to hypertension in certain susceptible people. There is evidence that taking birth control pills may be associated with hypertension in some women. Psychological and social factors—most notably stress—also seem to be involved, although the precise cause-and-effect relationship between stress and hypertension and the role that stress plays in the differentials between men and women need more extensive study. Women who drink 1 or 2 alcoholic beverages per day seem to be at lower risk for developing hypertension than those who drink nothing at all; women who drink heavily are at much higher risk.

Women who are obese—that is, who weigh at least 20 percent more than their ideal weight (see Weight Control)—develop hypertension 4 times more frequently than nonobese women of similar background. White women who are obese are 8 times more likely to develop high blood pressure, and 10 times more likely to have heart disease, than other women. Losing weight seems to be a good way to lower blood pressure.

The link between diabetes and high blood pressure is equally complicated. Not only are women with diabetes at increased risk for developing hypertension, but hypertension can also exacerbate the complications of diabetes. In addition, both hypertension and diabetes tend to occur together with high levels of blood fats and with obesity, both of which are risk factors for atherosclerosis and heart disease.

Other factors, such as smoking cigarettes, seem to increase the risk of complications once hypertension sets in. Serious complications of hypertension (such as kidney failure) are more likely to develop in African Americans than in people of other ethnic backgrounds. Whether this is because their hypertension is more severe or because there are differences in the arteries themselves is still unclear. Other factors such as differences in the sodium content of the diet, social stressors, lifestyle (especially exercise), and access to medical care may also help explain the disparate nature and rate of hypertension among people of different racial backgrounds.

Secondary hypertension tends to develop in women with various underlying conditions, including atherosclerosis, hyperthyroidism, hypothyroidism, Cushing syndrome, and, most commonly, kidney disorders. In the case of kidney disease, it is not always easy to know if the hypertension is primary or secondary, since high blood pressure can be either the cause or the effect of kidney disease.

If blood pressure is already high before pregnancy, it often rises even more during pregnancy. If hypertension develops after the 20th week, it can be a sign of preeclampsia—a serious condition that requires close monitoring by a clinician. Women who had hypertension before they became pregnant are considered to be at high risk for complications, and their fetuses are at risk for low birth weight. With good prenatal care and tight control of blood pressure, however, women prone to hypertension during pregnancy can usually deliver healthy, normal babies.

▸What are the symptoms?

Primary hypertension is a disease without symptoms. The only sure way to know that the blood vessels and organs are at risk for being damaged is a consistently high blood pressure reading.

Hypertension constricts the arterioles—the smallest and thinnest of the arteries throughout the body. One result can be an enlarged heart, since the heart muscle expands as it works more vigorously to pump blood into these vessels. As the heart enlarges, it begins to pump less effectively. In addition to causing heart disease, damage to arteries from high blood pressure can cause bleeding into the brain (a stroke) and into the retina of the eye (which can lead to blindness).

Heart attacks, congestive heart failure, stroke, and kidney disease occur because hypertension sets the stage for atherosclerosis—the process whereby blood vessels become clogged with fatty deposits and scar tissue.

If the clogged or blocked artery supplies blood to the heart, the result is chest pain (angina) and perhaps a heart attack. If the blocked artery supplies blood to the brain, the result may be a stroke. If it supplies blood to the kidney, the result can be kidney failure.

▸ How is the condition evaluated?

If a woman has elevated blood pressure on two separate occasions, a clinician will do a thorough physical examination to determine the extent of damage to the arteries, if any. Part of this examination will include a detailed family history of hypertension, hormonal abnormalities, and kidney disease, as well as a search for risk factors for heart disease. Various blood and urine tests (including a complete blood count and urinalysis) will also be performed to check the levels of glucose, cholesterol, triglycerides, uric acid, calcium, blood urea nitrogen (BUN), and creatinine. Sometimes an electrocardiogram will be done to evaluate heart rhythm. An ultrasound image can also indirectly give information about the effect of hypertension on the heart muscle.

In some cases a clinician may order additional tests to see if the problem is secondary hypertension (which occurs only 5 to 10 percent of the time). Indications for additional testing include hypertension that came on rapidly without any family history of the disease, or unusually severe and difficult-to-treat hypertension.

▸ How is high blood pressure treated?

Mild to moderate hypertension can often be controlled without resorting to medications. For example, weight reduction in an overweight woman is often enough to bring blood pressure down to normal. Women who are sodium-sensitive will find that their blood pressure responds to a low-sodium diet. Even for women who are not overweight, diet can be as effective as drugs for mild to moderate high blood pressure. A diet which includes 10 servings of fruits and vegetables a day, low-fat dairy products for protein, and a low-fat and low-salt intake achieves the same reduction in blood pressure as conventional drugs in the initial treatment of hypertension. If one drinks alcohol, limiting oneself to 7 drinks per week, cutting out cigarettes altogether, and increasing exercise may be helpful, although certain forms of exercise (such as lifting heavy weights) may actually increase blood pressure. If a woman with high blood pressure is taking oral contraceptives, her clinician may suggest that she stop taking them and switch to another form of birth control. Finally, biofeedback, stress management, meditation, and other relaxation techniques can be effective in some cases.

Women with suspected or known hypertension often find it helpful to purchase a blood pressure cuff to monitor their blood pressure at home. This allows more accurate assessment of average blood pressure than can be obtained with occasional readings done in the doctor's office. Simple equipment (a sphygmomanometer) is easy to use by the woman herself or with the help of a family member. Digital blood pressure cuffs can also be used, although the readings may not be quite as accurate.

When these lifestyle changes are unable to control hypertension, or when a woman is at high risk for complications, a clinician will prescribe one of several medications as well. Despite the prevalence (and, in the oldest age group, preponderance) of hypertension among women, most studies of hypertensive medications have involved only men. As a result, there is considerable controversy today about whether drugs routinely prescribed for this condition are as effective in women as in men, and whether they have comparable side effects.

Until more studies are done, however, women with otherwise uncontrollable hypertension should continue to use the same drugs men take. Among the most effective and best tolerated are ACE inhibitors, beta blockers, diuretics (water pills), and calcium-channel blockers. Although all these medications control high blood pressure extremely well, only ACE inhibitors and beta blockers have been proven to decrease the odds of a hypertension-related death from a heart attack. Just which drug is appropriate can vary according to a woman's race or overall health status. African American women, for example, generally respond better to diuretics or calcium-channel blockers than to beta blockers or ACE inhibitors.

Many other medications (such as hydralazine, aldomet, prazosin, and clonidine) can control high blood pressure, but they must be taken 2 to 4 times per day, and they produce more potential side effects than diuretics, beta blockers, calcium-channel blockers, and ACE inhibitors. But no matter which drugs are chosen, none is a cure for primary hypertension. It is vital for anyone with high blood pressure to keep taking medications for as long as they are prescribed—which often means for a lifetime. Because hypertension has no symptoms, many people stop taking their medications whenever they feel relatively healthy. Once the drugs are stopped, blood pressure rises again and eventually takes its toll on the arteries. And even when medications are taken faithfully, they are less effective in women who smoke, who are obese, and who do not get adequate exercise. Lifestyle changes in these areas can help lower blood pressure and decrease the risk of coronary artery disease.

If a woman needs more than 3 medications to control her blood pressure, a physician may advise testing for secondary causes of hypertension. Secondary hypertension is treated with some of the same drugs that are used for primary hypertension. If the underlying disease can be treated effectively, the associated hypertension will disappear as well.

Diuretics. These are the longest-studied and least expensive drugs for controlling high blood pressure. Also known as water or fluid pills, they seem to work by increasing the output of salt and water by the kidneys, thereby decreasing the volume of blood. Side effects are relatively minimal, generally limited to an increased frequency of urination. Occasionally fatigue or lightheadedness occurs. Anyone using diuretics needs occasional laboratory tests to check for chemical imbalances, especially low potassium, and a lipid profile.

ACE inhibitors. Angiotensin concerting enzyme inhibitors, including captopril (Capoten), enalapril (Vasotec), and lisinopril (Zestril, Prinivil), work by interfering with the production of a protein that constricts blood vessels. ACE inhibitors seem to cause even fewer side effects than some of the other antihypertensive medications and are one of the first-line therapies for hypertension. Occasional side effects include dry cough and in rare cases allergic reactions. ACE inhibitors are often preferable for the many women with diabetes as well as hypertension, since they do not have adverse effects on carbohydrate metabolism and seem to help preserve kidney function. These medications cannot be used during pregnancy because they cause birth defects.

Beta blockers. Propranolol (Inderal), metoprolol (Lopressor), and atenolol (Tenormin) are excellent medications for controlling high blood pressure and for preventing coronary artery disease. They work by blocking the blood vessels' ability to contract. Most patients notice no side effects from using beta blockers, especially the newer "cardioselective" ones such as atenolol. Among the possible side effects are slow pulse, fatigue, dizziness, diarrhea, cold or tingling fingers or toes, and dry mouth, eyes, or skin. Less often, people may develop insomnia, hallucinations, anxiety, confusion, depression, or breathing difficulties. Beta blockers should be used with caution by people with asthma.

Calcium-channel blockers. Verapamil (Calan, Isoptin), diltiazem (Cardizem), and nifedipine (Procardia, Adalat) reduce pressure in the arteries by preventing the entry of calcium into small blood vessels. Generally these drugs are well tolerated, but fatigue is an occasional side effect, and, less frequently, rapid heartbeat, dizziness, nausea, constipation, and swollen feet, ankles, or legs.

High Cholesterol

Cholesterol is an odorless, white, powdery chemical manufactured by the liver and used to make essential body substances such as cell walls and hormones. It is part of every animal cell and is found in all foods that come from animals. In the bloodstream (which transports cholesterol throughout the body), it is wrapped in protein "packages" called lipoproteins, which come in several forms. The lipoprotein that has been of greatest concern to investigators is low-density lipoprotein (LDL; sometimes referred to as "bad" cholesterol). This protein contains a high percentage of cholesterol relative to protein, and when LDL levels in the blood are high, cells lining the inside of the arteries transport LDL and its cholesterol load into the artery wall, setting the stage for atherosclerosis.

In atherosclerosis, scar tissue and fatty deposits build up in the walls of arteries throughout the body (see illustration). Eventually a clot can form on the surface of these obstructions, abruptly blocking the flow of blood in the already narrowed artery. If the blocked artery supplies blood to the heart, the result is chest pain (angina) and perhaps a heart attack.

Numerous studies in middle-aged men have linked high LDL levels in the blood to an increased risk of heart attacks, as well as stroke and other vascular diseases. They have also established that lowering LDL cholesterol in the blood reduces the risk of developing (and dying from) coronary artery disease (CAD). Whether these conclusions will turn out to be equally valid for premenopausal women—who, because of the presence of the hormone estrogen, seem to metabolize cholesterol differently—remains to be seen; several long-term investigations are currently addressing that question.

Preliminary evidence already suggests some important differences between men and women when it comes to cholesterol. For example, in women high levels of LDL in the blood seem not to be the best predictor of the risk of dying from cardiovascular disease and stroke, as they are in men. Rather, it is the level of HDL (high-density lipoprotein); women with higher levels of HDL seem to have less coronary artery disease. This "good" cholesterol contains a high

From cholesterol to coronary artery disease

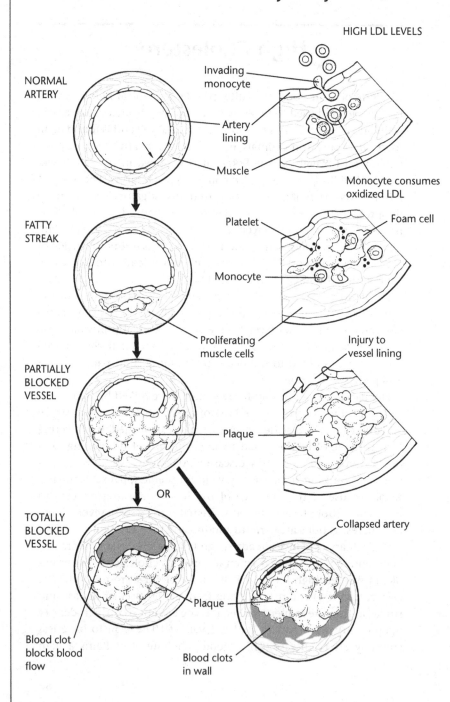

The cells lining healthy arteries protect them from damaging substances in the bloodstream. When LDL levels are high, these cells transport LDL into the artery wall, where—no longer protected by antioxidants in the blood—it oxidizes.

 Monocytes (white blood cells that repair injured tissue) consume the now-toxic LDL and swell to become foam cells. These appear as a fatty streak on the surface of the artery wall. In response, muscle cells proliferate, making the wall thicker. Platelets (blood-clotting elements in the blood) make growth factors that increase the thickening, which eventually becomes artherosclerotic plaque.

 Over decades, further injury to the artery lining from high blood pressure, toxic gases in cigarette smoke, or other factors causes scarring and the accumulation of debris, furthering narrowing the artery.

 Ultimately, a blood clot can form on the surface of the plaque or blood can leak into its core. In either event, the result can be a life-threatening blockage of blood flow to a vital artery.

percentage of protein relative to cholesterol and is believed to take cholesterol *away* from cells and transport it back to the liver for processing or removal.

Also, there is some preliminary evidence that, in women, having high triglyceride levels *combined with* low levels of HDL may be the most potent predictor of risk for CAD. Triglycerides are other lipids (fatlike substances) in the blood that are packaged in a third type of lipoprotein called VLDLs (very low density lipoproteins). Triglycerides seem to be less important as a predictor of risk in men.

Most people's blood cholesterol levels are relatively constant regardless of how much actual cholesterol they eat, since a feedback mechanism slows synthesis of cholesterol in the liver whenever dietary levels are high. But for the 1 person in 5 with a faulty mechanism of cholesterol control, changing cholesterol in the diet is the first line of defense against high blood levels of LDL. And since it is hard to know just which people have a defect in this mechanism, everyone has been advised by the National Institutes of Health (NIH) to limit dietary cholesterol to under 300 mg per day.

Today most people are aware that fats and oils, rather than cholesterol itself, are the major components of the diet that can raise LDL cholesterol to dangerous levels. Saturated fats, which come from animal tissues and some kinds of vegetable oils, in particular stimulate production of LDL relative to HDL. Because of the large toll taken by heart disease in the United States—and despite uncertainties about the meaning of high or low cholesterol levels in women (not to mention in the elderly of both sexes and in children)—the National Cholesterol Education Panel (NCEP) of the NIH has recommended that all people keep their intake of dietary fats and oils low.

More and better data may one day refine the NCEP's dietary and blood cholesterol recommendations for particular groups. It is known, for example, that estrogen alters the way women convert dietary cholesterol and fats into blood cholesterol, and this may help explain why premenopausal women (and those postmenopausal women who are taking estrogen replacement therapy) have a relatively low incidence of coronary artery disease, regardless of what they eat. But for the time being, the NCEP recommends that women and men of all ages strive for low blood cholesterol, and if necessary adjust their diet to accomplish that goal. Avoiding fried foods and eating skinless poultry, fish, shellfish, lean red meats, and low-fat dairy products, as well as ample portions of fruits and vegetables, breads and grains, and dried beans, are the first steps usually recommended.

▸ How is blood cholesterol evaluated?

The current NCEP screening guidelines recommend that all adults over the age of 20 have total cholesterol and HDL levels measured once every 5 years (total cholesterol is the combination of LDL and HDL). Since most of the total in both men and women consists of LDL, a high total cholesterol level generally indicates a high LDL level. Many doctors prefer to check levels at least twice, and to make sure that the two results are reasonably consonant, before drawing definitive conclusions. This is because cholesterol testing can be inaccurate, with wide discrepancies sometimes occurring between levels measured on different days or by different laboratories. Most often, if the first test shows high levels, a second will be done after a 12-hour fast. Generally more accurate results come from tests done on blood drawn from a vein in the arm as opposed to blood drawn from a finger.

The NCEP considers a total cholesterol of 200 mg/dL or less in the initial screening as desirable, 200 to 239 mg/dL as borderline high risk, and over 240 as high risk. Anyone who falls into the borderline-high or high-risk categories, as well as people in the low-risk category but who have HDL levels under 35 mg/dL, should have a more specific lipoprotein analysis to determine actual levels of LDL. This more specific test is performed after fasting for 9 to 12 hours, with two measurements taken from 1 to 8 weeks apart. Triglycerides are measured along with lipoproteins. If triglyceride levels are too high, the LDL measurement is considered inaccurate. The NCEP recommends this more detailed test as the initial screening procedure in people who already know they have coronary artery disease and in women with diabetes.

For people without preexisting coronary artery disease, LDL levels under 130 mg/dL are considered desirable, 130 mg/dL to 159 mg/dL are considered to be borderline high risk, and over 160 mg/dL is high risk. The NCEP recommends dietary changes for people in the high-risk group, as well as for people in the borderline-high group who also have two or more additional risk factors for coronary artery disease. These might include premature menopause, being over the age of 55 and not taking estrogen replacement therapy (ERT), having a family history of early coronary artery disease, smoking, having high blood pressure, and being obese or diabetic. (Diabetes in women erases any protection against coronary artery disease they get from being female, and in fact puts them in the highest-risk group.) These people should also have a complete physical examination, history, and laboratory tests to determine if some other condition (such as a hereditary disorder, hypothyroidism, or kidney disorders) may underlie the high lipid levels. If so, the NCEP dietary guidelines should be followed in addition to whatever other treatment is appropriate.

For people with preexisting coronary artery disease and women with diabetes, the NCEP recommends starting dietary therapy if LDL levels are between 100 and 130 mg/dL, and drug therapy if LDL is 130 mg/dL or higher.

▸ How is high cholesterol treated?

Dietary therapy. For people whose total blood cholesterol levels are too high, the NCEP recommends a 2-step dietary plan. In step 1, the diet should contain no more than 8 to 10 percent of calories from saturated fat, no more than 18 to 20 percent from other fats, and no more than 300 milligrams of cholesterol per day. In step 2, the daily diet should contain less than 7 percent of calories from saturated fat and less than 200 mg from cholesterol. For people trying to obliterate preexisting arterial plaque, an even more rigorous diet consisting of under 10 percent of calories from fat and 5 to 10 mg of cholesterol per day is recommended—a diet which few people are able to follow.

Overweight people are advised to lose weight, since this not only lowers LDL and triglyceride levels but also reduces hypertension, another risk factor for coronary artery disease. Combining weight reduction with physical exercise (and cooking with olive oil, a monounsaturate, which seems to have a beneficial effect on coronary risk) is also generally believed to decrease LDLs and triglycerides and increase HDLs.

Reducing saturated fat and cholesterol intake may lower HDL as well as LDL levels in women—and HDLs are thought to be important in protecting women from coronary artery disease. Adding regular exercise to the "heart-healthy" diet, however, seems to counter this reduction, bringing the HDLs back to the same level where they were before the beginning of the diet and exercise regime. Although lowering LDLs is supposed to be beneficial for everyone, the fact that HDL levels are better predictors of a woman's risk of coronary artery disease leaves in question the overall benefit of a diet that might lower HDL at the same time that it lowers LDL. Still, at present, in light of the great uncertainty, most doctors recommend that women generally follow the NCEP's guidelines—with special attention to HDL levels.

As with all recommendations about cholesterol, however, women should take dietary guidelines with a grain of salt. For one thing, current beliefs about the exact effect of specific dietary fats on cholesterol levels are in a state of flux and are bound to change as better information accumulates. New data keep pouring in, making it clear that original proclamations about good and bad foods were far too simplistic. No longer are all saturated fats considered alike. For example, though 3 of the 4 types of saturated fat do appear to raise total blood cholesterol levels, the type found in beef and chocolate (called stearic acid) is now considered neutral. Similarly, while monounsaturated fats (such as those in olive oil) have been touted as desirable alternatives to saturated fats, it appears that one structural form of monounsaturates (found in margarine and many packaged snack foods) actually increases the risk of coronary artery disease in women.

Although polyunsaturated fats such as those found in fish oils may decrease the blood's ability to clot and therefore decrease the risk of heart attacks and stroke, they are also easily incorporated into LDLs and may make them more susceptible to oxidation, which promotes atherosclerosis. A few studies have suggested an increased risk of cancer from a diet that contains more than 10 percent polyunsaturated fats, while others have suggested that polyunsaturates can lower HDL levels as well as LDL levels—and this is not desirable. The American Heart Association advises limiting polyunsaturated fats to 10 percent of caloric intake.

Significantly altering blood cholesterol levels through diet alone can require considerable effort and change in lifestyle. The success of a given diet varies with the individual, but the average person can anticipate that following the NCEP's guidelines will reduce LDL and total cholesterol by 10 to 15 percent. This means that a person who starts out with a total cholesterol count of 300 can reasonably expect to lower it to only about 260 by diet alone. A person who starts with a total cholesterol level of 220 can expect to lower it to about 195.

It usually takes at least 6 months, with nutritional consultation, for LDL levels to fall. If they fail to fall after this amount of time, drug therapy may be necessary.

Drug therapy. Because low levels of HDL may be an important risk factor for coronary artery disease in women, many clinicians recommend drug therapy both to reduce LDL and to increase HDL if dietary therapy is ineffective. Most of the anticholesterol drugs, with the exception of niacin, decrease LDL but do not increase HDL. Some even decrease HDL. Unless there is a family history of high cholesterol or additional risk factors for CAD, drugs are generally not prescribed as the first line of therapy for premenopausal women. In addition, there is still no general agreement about the best treatment for women who have normal LDLs, low HDLs, and borderline-high to high triglyceride levels. At the moment many experts suggest that such patients should try to increase physical activity and, when appropriate, reduce weight.

There are 5 main categories of cholesterol-lowering drugs: bile acid sequestrants, 3-hydroxy-3-methylglutaryl coenzyme A (HMG Co A) reductase inhibitors, nicotinic acid, fibric acid derivatives, and probucol.

The bile acid sequestrants—which include cholestyramine (Questran) and colestipol (Colestid)—are usually prescribed to people with high LDL levels. They work by lowering these levels and slightly increasing HDL levels. Side effects can include constipation, abdominal pain, nausea, and bloating.

The 3 HMG Co A reductase inhibitors (such as lovastatin and pravastatin, sold under the trade names Mevacor and Pravachol) also work by lowering LDL levels and slightly increasing HDLs, but they are sometimes associated with a different set of side effects—including hepatitis and muscle inflammation. They are not given to pregnant women or women considering pregnancy because of the risk of birth defects.

People with high LDL and triglyceride levels and low HDL levels may be prescribed nicotinic acid (niacin), which lowers LDLs and triglycerides and raises HDLs. Niacin is a naturally occurring vitamin found in many foods, but at therapeutic doses it can occasionally result in side effects, including hepatitis, gout, hyperglycemia, ulcer formation, insomnia, various skin disorders, and certain heart arrhythmias (irregular heartbeat). Taking an aspirin half an hour before a dose of niacin and taking it with meals can lessen unpleasant flushing.

Another category of drugs, fibric acid derivatives such as clofibrate (Atromid) and gemfibrozil (Lopid) lowers triglycerides, raises HDLs, and either raises or lowers LDLs. Side effects may include gallstones, hepatitis, high LDL levels, decreased sex drive, muscle inflammation, heart arrhythmias, increased appetite, abdominal pain, and nausea.

The fifth category of lipid-lowering drugs consists of the drug probucol (Lorelco), which is generally prescribed to people with an inherited form of high cholesterol. Besides lowering both LDL and HDL levels, probucol functions as a potent antioxidant—that is, it prevents oxidation, which is thought to prompt LDLs to promote atherosclerosis. Side effects can include altered heart rhythms, low HDL levels, diarrhea, bloating, nausea, and abdominal pain.

Any of the lipid-lowering drugs can reduce blood cholesterol levels by as much as 30 percent within 6 weeks. In addition, some researchers are now suggesting that antioxidants, such as vitamin E, may prove beneficial by preventing the formation of oxidized forms of LDLs. Anyone taking cholesterol-lowering medications should have blood lipid levels checked regularly.

Estrogen replacement therapy. Another drug therapy particularly relevant to postmenopausal women is estrogen replacement therapy. Women taking ERT have lower levels of LDL, higher levels of HDL, and lower rates of coronary artery disease than women the same age not on ERT. Although estrogen replacement may mildly increase triglyceride levels, this is usually a problem only if a woman has abnormally high triglyceride levels before starting ERT.

All of these effects on cholesterol levels and triglycerides result only from estrogens taken by mouth, which are metabolized in the liver. The patch form, which delivers estrogen through the skin directly into the bloodstream, apparently has no effect on lipid levels (see Estrogen Replacement Therapy).

Whether or not these effects are as great in women using combination therapy (both estrogen and progesterone, currently the most common form of hormone replacement therapy) remains to be seen. Progesterone increases LDL levels and decreases HDLs, but the data available so far suggest that adding progesterone does not significantly undermine the beneficial effects of estrogen on a woman's coronary risk. The final verdict will have to wait until results are in from the large-scale randomized trials currently being conducted as part of the NIH-sponsored Women's Health Initiative.

Obesity

Obesity means an excess of total body fat. In the past a woman was considered obese if she weighed at least 20 percent more than her ideal weight. It is quite possible, however, for a person to exceed the ideal weight for her height and still not have excess body fat if the weight of her bones and muscles is unusually high. In general, however, people who are significantly overweight also tend to be obese, which explains why the two terms are frequently used interchangeably.

In the United States 27 percent of women and 24 percent of men between the ages of 20 and 74 weigh more than they should, according to standard height-weight charts (see Weight Control). But as many as 40 percent of all American women claim to be "dieting" or actively engaged in some kind of weight control program. Study after study seems to confirm that the vast majority of them will fail in their efforts (necessary or not) to lose weight over the long haul.

▸ Who is likely to be obese?

Obesity occurs when a person takes in more energy (in the form of food) than she uses up (by burning calories during physical activity); the excess energy gets stored as fat. But why some people are more prone to such an imbalance remains unclear. Overeating certainly has something to do with obesity, but some people seem to be able to eat everything in sight and stay at their ideal weight; others gain weight on very low calorie regimens.

Genetics certainly plays a role: if one parent is obese, each child has a 40 percent chance of also being obese. And if both parents are obese, the risk to each child rises to 80 percent. Overweight children and adolescents are more likely than others to become obese adults. Both genetic and cultural factors are thought to explain the higher prevalence of obesity in African American and Hispanic women, who do not seem to be as obsessed with thinness as white women are. For example, in a recent survey 64 percent of black teenage girls said it was better to be a little overweight than a little underweight;

by contrast, the majority of white teenage girls in the survey claimed that they would "rather be dead than fat."

Both men and women are more likely to become overweight as they age. In men the peak incidence of obesity occurs between the ages of 45 and 54, whereas in women the peak incidence is between 65 and 74, when they are generally at their most sedentary and least inclined or able to undertake regular physical exercise.

▸ How is the condition evaluated?

In recent years sophisticated measures of body fat have begun to be used in conjunction with weight to determine if a woman is obese. One of these measures is called the body mass index (BMI), which indicates how much of the weight comes from muscle or bone versus fat. It is calculated by multiplying weight in pounds by 700 and then dividing the product by the square of height in inches. That means that a woman who weighs 125 pounds and stands 5'5" (65 inches) tall would have a BMI of $(125 \times 700)/(65 \times 65)$ or about 21. A BMI higher than 25 is considered to be reason for concern. Therefore, a 5'5" woman weighing 170 pounds would have a BMI of $(170 \times 700)/(65 \times 65)$ or about 28 and would be labeled obese by this measure.

Another useful measure of obesity is waist-to-hip ratio, calculated by measuring the smallest area around the waist (with the stomach relaxed) and then dividing this number by the measurement of the widest area around the hips. A waist-to-hip ratio greater than 0.8 in women aged 40 to 59 has been associated with elevated risk for diabetes, high blood pressure, and gallbladder disease (see illustration).

To determine both the causes and the effects of a patient's obesity, the physician will ask questions about the presence of any medical conditions, as well as the history of dieting and physical activity. Often some routine biochemical and metabolic tests will be performed to check for physiological problems, and overall physical fitness will be evaluated.

In addition to diabetes and high blood pressure, both of which are linked to an increased risk of coronary artery disease, obesity is also associated with osteoarthritis of the spine, endometrial cancer (because fat produces estrogen, an excess of which can stimulate abnor-

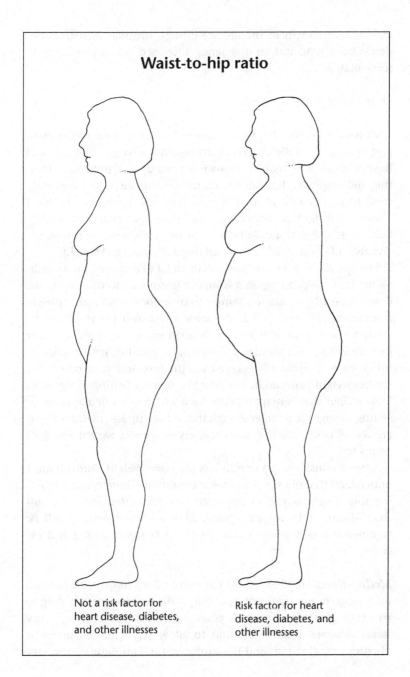

Waist-to-hip ratio

Not a risk factor for
heart disease, diabetes,
and other illnesses

Risk factor for heart
disease, diabetes, and
other illnesses

mal cellular growth in the uterine lining), irregular menstruation, excess body hair, and, in pregnancy, increased risk of preeclampsia (toxemia).

▸ How is obesity treated?

Diet and exercise. Dieting is a national pastime among women, in part because most dieters eventually regain the weight they lost and have to go on another diet. Many even end up weighing more than they did originally. But this should not discourage people who truly need to lose weight from trying. In fact, many people who were obese lose weight by focusing on realistic weight goals and healthy behaviors. The goal should be to improve or alleviate the symptoms and risks of obesity rather than striving for some ideal weight.

The specific weight loss plan needs to be determined on an individual basis, depending on a woman's history, concerns, and goals. One reason why so many attempts to treat obesity fail is that people assume that all obesity has the same cause and therefore can be treated in the same way. For one woman successful treatment may involve losing a set number of pounds; for another, merely stabilizing a yo-yo pattern of repeated weight loss and gain or halting further weight gain can be considered a success. Setting as a goal an ideal weight that is inappropriate for a woman's particular body, or setting a weight loss target so high that achieving and maintaining it are too difficult, are the main reasons why most weight loss programs fail.

Anyone considering a weight loss plan (see Weight Control) must understand that obesity is a chronic condition. Therefore, maintaining lost weight is just as important as—and often more difficult than—losing it in the first place. Almost always, weight will be regained unless a woman changes her patterns of eating and exercise.

Medications. In 1996 the FDA approved dexfenfluramine (Redux) for long-term management of obesity—the first weight loss drug to win FDA approval in over 20 years. Around the same time, many states loosened their regulations to allow physicians to prescribe phentermine (Ioamin) and DL-fenfluramine (Pondimin) for weight

loss. The new availability of drug therapy for obesity is revolutioniz-
ing the medical approach to this condition for some women.

Drug therapy for obesity is not a magic bullet, however. It has a
relatively modest effect on weight loss (5 to 10 pounds beyond what
can be achieved with diet and exercise alone). Because these drugs
work primarily by reducing carbohydrate craving, weight is often
regained after stopping the drugs, requiring that they be used off
and on for several years. As yet very little is known about the safety
of weight loss medications taken long-term.

Two forms of drug therapy are currently in use: dexfenfluramine
(sold under the brand name Redux) and a combination of some
form of fenfluramine with phentermine (popularly known as fen-
phen and available generically). Although the effectiveness of the
two regimens is fairly similar, Redux, because it is not available in
generic form, is more expensive (approximately $2 per day). Redux
has been approved by the FDA for up to one year of use, and only in
people whose weight poses a significant health risk. Fen-phen combinations are FDA-approved for only 3 to 6 months of use.

It is clear, however, that some unscrupulous physicians and
weight loss centers are providing prescriptions to people who are
only slightly overweight, and are unnecessarily exposing them to a
rare but life-threatening complication: pulmonary hypertension.
The risk rises from about 1 to about 18 in a million after 3 months of
drug use. To put this risk into perspective, drug companies have
estimated that for every death from pulmonary hypertension, 28
lives could be saved by reducing the risk of death from complications related to obesity.

To determine whether drug therapy is appropriate for an individual woman, a physician should consider her weight loss history, the
presence of medical conditions that are aggravated by obesity (such
as high blood pressure, arthritis, heart disease, or diabetes), and her
degree of overweight. Drug therapy may be appropriate if her BMI is
more than 30 (about 30 percent above desirable weight) or, when
there are other risk factors, more than 27 (about 20 percent above
desirable weight). Women who are pregnant, nursing, or taking
certain antidepressants (MAO inhibitors or SSRIs) must not take
these weight loss drugs.

If, after weighing all the risks and benefits, a woman and her physician choose drug therapy for obesity, it is important that her clinician regularly monitor her response to the drugs and watch for side effects: loose stools or diarrhea, dry mouth, and drowsiness from fenfluramine; jitteriness, headache, and elevation of blood pressure from phentermine. Side effects can sometimes be eliminated by adjusting the dosage.

Surgery. As a last resort surgery may be considered, particularly if a woman has 100 pounds or more to lose. The two most commonly performed procedures aim at making it impossible to eat large amounts of food by shortening the amount of time it takes for food to get from the stomach to the small intestine. In the older and riskier of these two procedures, gastric bypass, most of the stomach is closed and reconnected to the small intestine. The second procedure, gastroplasty, is somewhat less effective but has fewer complications. Here the surgeon makes a small vertical passageway from the stomach to the small intestine by closing off the upper third of the stomach with sutures or staples.

With either procedure the patient can expect to lose approximately half her excess weight within the first year, although loss slows in the second year, and some weight may be regained after that. Few patients ever lose all their excess weight through surgery alone. Side effects and complications can include nausea, vomiting, and, over the long term, nutrient deficiencies (especially of vitamin B_{12}, folic acid, and iron).

Women who have had weight loss surgery are advised to postpone pregnancy until their weight has stabilized for a year or two. Once a woman becomes pregnant, she will need to be monitored carefully to make sure that she gains weight and that nutrition is adequate for the developing fetus.

Stroke

A stroke is one of several potentially fatal disorders that occur after the blood supply to the brain is disturbed. Although strokes happen more frequently in men than in women after age 30, women who have strokes are twice as likely to die of them. This may be because women have a longer life expectancy and tend to have strokes at later ages. In addition, certain conditions unique to or more common in females—such as pregnancy and mitral valve prolapse (the ballooning out of the valve linking the upper and lower chambers of the heart)—may predispose certain women to strokes.

Strokes fall into two basic categories depending on the cause: infarcts and cerebral hemorrhages.

Infarcts. These are similar to heart attacks in that some of the brain's nerve tissue dies when its blood supply is reduced. Like coronary artery disease, infarcts result most often from atherosclerosis, a condition in which arteries are clogged with fatty deposits and scar tissue that eventually enlarge and harden into plaque. In people with atherosclerosis, a blood clot (thrombus) may form in the narrowed channel and block blood flow to the brain, a condition called cerebral thrombosis. In other cases, called cerebral embolism, a piece of plaque or a blood clot dislodges from the heart or a blood vessel and travels to block the flow of blood in an artery supplying the brain.

Cerebral hemorrhage. Strokes in this category occur when an artery leaks blood into or around the brain, eventually resulting in tissue death. In women many strokes occur because an aneurysm (bulge) in an artery in the head ruptures.

▸ Who is likely to have a stroke?
The risk of having a stroke rises with age, with the chances doubling for each decade beyond the age of 35. Atherosclerosis, hypertension, diabetes, and smoking all increase the risk of stroke in both men and women.

83

Certain inherited or acquired conditions can increase the likelihood of blood clots and therefore strokes. These conditions include cancer, immobilization in bed, and certain blood disorders, as well as the presence of antibodies in the blood that are sometimes found in women with lupus and certain blood abnormalities. In addition, people who have already had temporary deficiencies in the blood supply to the brain (called transient ischemic attacks) owing to a narrowing of the small arteries in the brain circulation or of the larger carotid arteries in the neck are prone to strokes.

Certain forms of heart disease such as a recent heart attack, deformities of the heart valves, or heart rhythm problems (called atrial fibrillation; see illustration) are associated with embolic strokes. In younger women with mitral valve prolapse (which is 3 times more common in women than in men), the risk of stroke rises fourfold—although because a young woman's chances of having a stroke are so low in the first place, even a fourfold rise means the risk of having a stroke is still quite low. Abnormally high cholesterol levels, obesity, and migraine headaches have been linked to strokes, but more studies need to be done before these links are clearly established.

Hemorrhagic strokes are a rare complication of pregnancy, but they remain a leading cause of maternal death (which is also rare). Pregnant women often have increased coagulability of the blood and may develop blood clots or emboli during the last trimester of pregnancy. The increased cardiac output and blood volume in the second and third trimesters of pregnancy may lead to the rupture of preexisting aneurysms. Even more rarely eclampsia in a pregnant woman may lead to stroke, as may significant blood loss during delivery.

Contrary to earlier belief, there is no convincing evidence that using oral contraceptives increases most women's risk of stroke. Even so, many doctors advise women who smoke, abuse substances such as cocaine or amphetamines, or have a history of blood clots to use oral contraceptives cautiously.

▸ What are the symptoms?

Symptoms of a stroke, as well as its long-term effects, depend on how much and which parts of the brain are affected. Common

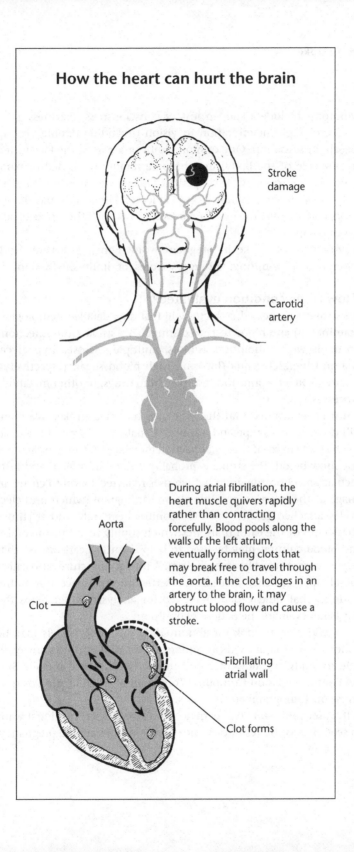

How the heart can hurt the brain

Stroke damage

Carotid artery

During atrial fibrillation, the heart muscle quivers rapidly rather than contracting forcefully. Blood pools along the walls of the left atrium, eventually forming clots that may break free to travel through the aorta. If the clot lodges in an artery to the brain, it may obstruct blood flow and cause a stroke.

Aorta

Clot

Fibrillating atrial wall

Clot forms

symptoms include a sudden loss of consciousness, dizziness, confusion, or rapid deterioration in vision (including double vision), speech, or sensation. One or more limbs or a part of the face (often on one side of the body) may become rapidly weakened or paralyzed. The person may also experience headache, vomiting, or difficulty in swallowing. Symptoms last at least 24 hours but may fluctuate in severity over the first day or two, after which the stroke is said to be "complete."

Symptoms of stroke in pregnant women include severe headaches, nausea, vomiting, lethargy, seizures, or diminished vision.

▸ How is the condition evaluated?

If a stroke is suspected, a doctor will first do a detailed neurological examination and blood tests to distinguish a stroke from infections (treatable with antibiotics), tumors, multiple sclerosis, hypoglycemia and hyperglycemia (low and high blood sugar, respectively), seizures, sudden confusion resulting from drugs, or other metabolic processes.

If it is determined that the woman is having a stroke, treatment will depend on its type and location. Usually a CT scan of the head will be done to see if there has been hemorrhage. If the CT scan does not show blood, the stroke is probably due to an infarct, and tests such as an echocardiogram (which uses reflected sound to create an image of the heart), a portable electrocardiogram (which uses electrodes attached to the body to monitor heart rate and rhythm), ultrasound of the carotid arteries which supply blood to the brain, and blood cultures may be used to help identify heart disease that might have resulted in an embolism. A lumbar puncture (also called spinal tap)—in which a needle is inserted into the space around the spine so that fluid can be removed for analysis—often helps the physician evaluate the patient's condition.

An MRI scan to look for abnormalities in blood vessels may be done; and in major medical centers, new radiologic tests are available to study the flow of blood in the brain. These include Single Photon Emission Computed Tomography (SPECT) and Positron Emission Tomography (PET) scans.

If a pregnant woman experiences a stroke, a doctor will first want to see if it was the result of some condition unrelated to pregnancy.

She will usually be evaluated with an MRI or CT scan and, if necessary, an angiogram—an x-ray lasting 1 to 3 hours in which injected dye allows a doctor to see blood circulating within the vessels of the brain. To protect the developing fetus from the hazards of radiation, the pelvic area is shielded.

▸ How is stroke treated?

Emergency treatment for a person having a stroke involves calling an ambulance and having the person lie down, with any paralyzed parts protected from movement. No food or drink should be given, and if vomiting occurs, the woman's head should be turned to one side. If she has difficulty breathing, it may help to raise her head and shoulders; if breathing stops completely, cardiopulmonary resuscitation (CPR) should be started. Except in the case of extremely mild strokes involving a day or two of weakness or dizziness, most people who have had a stroke will need to be admitted to the hospital. Often intensive care may be required to maintain basic functions.

Although no drug can revive dead nerve tissue, certain medications can prevent further damage. Certain patients may be candidates for thrombolytic therapy (see Coronary Artery Disease). For women whose strokes are not due to hemorrhage and who do not have high blood pressure, simply taking one aspirin tablet per day seems to be quite effective in reducing the risk of subsequent strokes. This is probably because aspirin inhibits blood clotting; often a cause of stroke is a blood clot that gets stuck in an artery already partially obstructed by plaque. Studies so far have involved mostly men, however, and there is some evidence that aspirin, at least in higher doses, is more effective in men than in women.

If a woman using aspirin continues to have stroke symptoms or cannot tolerate the side effects, the drug ticlopidine (Ticlid) is sometimes used. Like aspirin, Ticlid inhibits the blood's ability to clot. In a few women, however, this drug may cause a severe reduction in certain forms of white blood cells, so anyone using it must have blood counts done regularly, at least at the beginning of treatment.

Sometimes surgery is required to remove blood from brain tissues after a hemorrhagic stroke or to correct an underlying aneurysm.

Pregnant women who have had strokes are usually treated with bed rest, plenty of fluids, and drugs that prevent subsequent convulsions and blood clotting. About a quarter of strokes during pregnancy result in death; survival depends on where the stroke occurs and the degree of damage. If the damaged area is limited, there may be few lasting effects.

Physical, occupational, or speech therapy is often essential after a woman has had a stroke. These programs can help educate patients and their families about stroke and teach prevention of common complications such as limb contractures and bedsores. Physical therapy, including speech therapy, can sometimes help "train" other areas of the brain to take over functions once performed by the dead tissue. To be most effective, rehabilitation therapy should be started as soon as possible after the stroke.

▸ How can strokes be prevented?

Preventing stroke involves eliminating or reducing as many risk factors as possible. Avoiding cigarette smoking and normalizing blood pressure offer the biggest payoff in stroke prevention. In women with a history of certain forms of heart disease, the risk of embolic stroke can be reduced with long-term anticoagulation therapy. This usually involves taking a drug called warfarin (Coumadin). Women with severely narrowed carotid arteries can also reduce their risk of stroke or its recurrence through the surgical removal of plaque. A large recent study indicates, however, that women are less likely than men to benefit from this surgery. Researchers at the National Institute of Neurological Disorders and Stroke (NINDS) are trying to determine why this is so.

Pregnant women with heart failure or irregular heartbeat (arrhythmia) should be treated with bed rest, digoxin (a heart drug), and diuretics (pills that increase the volume of the urine and keep blood pressure down). Drugs that reduce the coagulability of the blood may also be necessary. The anticoagulant with the least risk to the fetus is heparin, which does not cross the placenta.

Taking Control

Alcohol Use

In the last decade or so considerable controversy has arisen about whether women who drink moderate amounts of alcohol might actually be healthier than either nondrinkers or heavy drinkers. Until recently the evidence in favor of alcohol came largely from studies on men, and it indicated that drinking 2 alcoholic beverages a day significantly reduces deaths from clogged heart arteries—probably because alcohol increases levels of high-density (HDL) cholesterol and reduces the formation of plaque in blood vessels. (These findings, in turn, fed speculations about the "French paradox": perhaps it was the red wine along with meals that explained why the French, with their cream-laden cuisine, were not unusually prone to heart disease.)

Most clinicians hesitated to extend these findings to women, however, partly because women are known to metabolize alcohol somewhat differently than men (accumulating more alcohol in their blood more readily) and partly because women who drink may be particularly susceptible to alcoholic liver disease and breast cancer.

It now appears that light to moderate drinking may indeed decrease deaths from all causes in women over the age of 50. A major 12-year study of 86,000 nurses aged 34 to 59 (part of the ongoing Harvard Nurses' Health Study) showed that women over 50 who drank between 1 and 20 drinks per week had a lower risk of death, particularly from cardiovascular disease, than nondrinkers. Heavier drinking (more than 20 drinks per week) was associated with an increased risk of death from other causes, particularly cirrhosis and breast cancer. (One drink = 12 ounces of beer = 5 ounces of wine = 1.5 ounces of 80-proof liquor. All of these are equivalent to 0.5 ounces or 12 grams of ethanol.)

The benefits were greatest for women who were at risk for heart disease—for example, women who were obese, smoked cigarettes, or had high cholesterol levels, high blood pressure, diabetes, or a family history of heart disease. Women 34 to 39 years of age who drank had a slightly higher risk of death from all causes regardless of how much they drank, but the number of deaths in this group was small.

▸ To drink or not to drink

This large and convincing study did not suggest that a nondrinker who suddenly adds a few drinks to her diet will necessarily lower her risk of cardiovascular disease. The benefits appeared only in women over 50 who were already drinkers when the study began. As in all studies of this type, it is possible that the lower death rates were attributable not to alcohol per se but to some other (unknown) factor common among women who drink moderately over the course of their adult lives. The only way to know for sure that alcohol itself confers health benefits would be to conduct a prospective study in which a group of nondrinkers started to drink moderately and were compared over time to an otherwise similar group who continued to abstain. Such a study seems unlikely.

If one adds to this research limitation the fact that women under 50 and risk-free women in the study showed no benefit from moderate drinking, and the fact that heavy drinking substantially increases a woman's risk of death, it does not make sense for nondrinkers to start drinking alcohol for the sake of their health. But for those women who already drink in moderation, most experts believe that they can continue in good conscience.

Diet

Women are prone to a number of heart-related diseases that may stem from, or be exacerbated by, diet, such as coronary artery disease, diabetes, and high blood pressure.

The evidence accumulated in recent years has been impressive in suggesting links between the presence or absence of certain types of foods in the diet and a person's susceptibility to these diseases. For example, the amount and kinds of fat in the diet can affect blood levels of cholesterol, which in turn are associated with the risk of coronary artery disease. Extremely low fat intake over a lifetime is associated with a higher than normal risk of hemorrhagic stroke, whereas a diet high in fat seems to raise the risk of cardiovascular disease.

The temptation—especially for someone already at risk for one of these diseases—is to change dietary habits as soon as one of these results is announced. The extravagance with which nutritional claims are touted in the popular press, however, is not always proportional to the scientific evidence backing them up. Few nutritional studies to date can be considered conclusive; most of them merely provide intriguing clues about the complex relationships between different foods and human health. Most of the studies can only establish correlations rather than prove cause and effect, and do not account for a number of variables that undoubtedly play a role in human health and disease. Furthermore, since many nutrients interact with other nutrients in the diet, consuming large quantities of one type may cut down absorption of another—or may be ineffective without adequate intake of yet a third.

The fact that nutritional science is still in its infancy helps explain why nutrition has been so long neglected in medical schools and is often overlooked by physicians as a possible means of preventing and treating disease. It also helps explain the conflicting claims that so frequently appear in the popular press. The result of so much hype, on the one hand, has been a growing skepticism among some members of the American public, who have come to believe that nutritional "breakthroughs" are not worth the newsprint required to

Food pyramid

The U.S. Department of Agriculture recommends a daily diet that contains fewer foods from the top of this pyramid and more from the bottom.

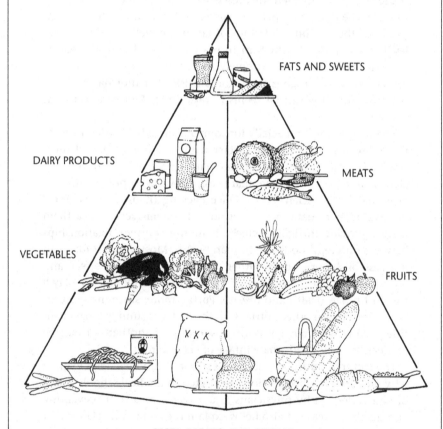

FATS AND SWEETS

DAIRY PRODUCTS

MEATS

VEGETABLES

FRUITS

PASTA, BREADS, AND CEREALS

announce them. On the other hand, because of media attention to nutrition, some people eagerly await the latest and presumably more accurate proclamation, assuming that there are easy, universal answers to the question, What should I eat?

▸ What do nutritional experts currently recommend?

Nutritional needs vary according to a person's age, sex, and reproductive status, and they also vary from individual to individual within those groups, depending on a person's unique genetic makeup and life situation. In an attempt to help people plan balanced diets that reflect current understanding of nutrition, in 1992 the U.S. Department of Agriculture replaced the traditional "four food groups" with the "Food Pyramid" (see illustration), a guide to daily food choices. Although it is based primarily on well-documented studies, it represents a certain amount of educated guessing, and it is not without its critics. Many of them contend that the Food Pyramid was shaped as much by the interests of the U.S. meat and dairy industries as by objective nutritional knowledge. A food pyramid put out by the government of a Mediterranean country, for example, would probably look quite different, perhaps increasing the recommended amount of olive oil and lowering the amount of milk and meat. Even so, most nutritionists laud the Food Pyramid's overall goal of increasing U.S. consumption of grains, fruits, and vegetables.

▸ Eating for a healthy heart

Because of the heavy toll taken by heart disease in the United States, and the many studies linking blood cholesterol levels with coronary artery disease, the National Cholesterol Education Panel (NCEP) of the National Institutes of Health recommends that Americans reduce their fat intake (from meats, dairy products, and all types of oils) to 30 percent or less of total calories, reduce saturated fats (primarily from meats and from some oils such as coconut oil) to less than 10 percent of total calories, and reduce cholesterol in the diet (from eggs, shrimp, and some other seafoods) to less than 300 mg daily. The American Heart Association, noting that polyunsaturated fats can lower levels of HDL (the "good" cholesterol), advises limiting polyunsaturated fats to 10 percent of caloric intake as well. Monounsaturated fats such as olive oil should make up the remaining 10 percent of daily caloric intake from fats and oils, since in some studies they seem to lower coronary risk.

Useful as all of these recommendations may be, they are still open to interpretation when it comes to planning individual meals. Should fat be reduced to 30 percent—or 20 percent—of the diet? Should red meat be avoided altogether? Will drinking more milk and eating more dairy products raise one's fat consumption and perhaps increase the risk of coronary artery disease? What are the pros and cons of refined sugar versus artificial sweeteners? What about salt? It is important to remember that there are no hard and fast answers to these questions.

Admonitions to cut back on calories, for example, or eliminate salt, or lower saturated fat intake do not necessarily apply to each individual woman. The recommended 2,100 calories a day can be perfectly fine for one woman, but it may lead another to gain unwanted pounds, while leaving a physically active woman constantly hungry. Although cutting down on salt does help lower blood pressure in some women, it has no effect on many others. And though some women's cholesterol levels do drop when they cut down on dietary cholesterol and saturated fats, many others compensate for this deprivation by producing more cholesterol in the liver. Dietary goals are blanket statements intended either to cover the widest segment of the population possible or to establish guidelines to protect the people most in need. These goals are not necessarily applicable to any one individual.

What makes sense, then, is for the individual woman to be aware of these general nutritional guidelines and then determine to the best of her ability if they seem to make sense for her, given her family and medical history, and her personal lifestyle. In general, there is little evidence that gorging on or abstaining from any one particular food or group of foods is enough to overcome the many other factors that predict human health and longevity—factors including genetics, family history, and one's living and working environment, as well as exercise and other behaviors related to lifestyle.

Despite these caveats, some diets are, in general, clearly more healthful than others. The challenge is making everyday decisions in the face of conflicting information. This can be accomplished to some extent by aiming to eat a balanced, varied diet and modifying it according to individual needs. A healthful diet is low in fat, moderate in protein, and high in complex carbohydrates. It includes relatively large amounts of vegetables, fruits, and grains and sparing use of fats, oils, and sugar.

After young adulthood, women's caloric needs gradually decline so that by menopause most women need only about two thirds of the calories they needed at the age of 20. Because decreased estrogen levels in the body seem to make women more susceptible to cardiovascular disorders, many nutritionists suggest that postmenopausal women restrict intake of fats, cholesterol, and possibly salt. Beyond that, women with heart disease, hypertension, or diabetes should consult their clinician about more specific dietary modifications. Because many medications can interfere with the body's absorption of nutrients, a clinician should also be consulted about any necessary supplementation.

▸ Coffee

For years coffee—or the stimulant in it, caffeine—has been suspected of causing heart disease and numerous other disorders. To the relief of those who enjoy sampling exotic blends or simply starting the day with a cup of instant Maxwell House, coffee has retained a relatively unblemished record despite all the outcry.

The evidence linking coffee or caffeine to cardiovascular disease remains unconvincing. A few studies have suggested that caffeine, at least in certain doses, may have some effect on blood cholesterol levels or on temporary rises in blood pressure. And some studies have suggested that drinking more than 3 or 4 cups of coffee a day may moderately increase the risk of having a heart attack—at least in men. These controversial studies have included both caffeinated and decaffeinated coffee. But other equally impressive studies have shown no such associations, so for now there is no reason to believe that moderate coffee consumption puts people at risk for cardiovascular disease.

Some of the health problems that have been attributed to coffee consumption may instead be due to other potentially harmful habits that tend to be more common in coffee drinkers—such as cigarette smoking, lack of exercise, or a higher than average amount of fat or alcohol in the diet.

All the same, caffeine is a mild stimulant drug that definitely has some clear-cut effects on the human body. It may increase levels of the stress hormone adrenalin in the body, and it can be responsible for an irregular or pounding heart beat.

Coffee is not the only culprit when it comes to caffeine. Plenty of other beverages—as well as various medications for insomnia, appetite control, and headaches—are sources of the stimulant, although, when it comes to beverages, coffee is indeed the most common source.

▸ Artificial sweeteners

There is no reason for most healthy people to fear the effects of moderate amounts of sugar in their diet. But sugar adds calories, and for people trying to lose weight, sugar can contribute to obesity. For them, as well as for people with diabetes (whose bodies metabolize sugar abnormally), artificial sweeteners may be a desirable way to enjoy otherwise forbidden foods.

Artificial sweeteners are heavily used in the United States, particularly by women. They can be found in diet soft drinks and many dietetic foods, and are sold for home consumption in supermarkets. Restaurant tables frequently include little packets of artificial sweetener alongside the regular sugar. It is therefore surprising that so little concrete evidence exists showing that artificial sweeteners actually help people lose weight. For the most part, artificial sweeteners simply allow people watching their weight to indulge in foods and drinks they would otherwise have to avoid. The downside of artificial sweeteners is that dieters using them may develop a false sense of security and end up overindulging in some other food.

Estrogen Replacement Therapy

Estrogen replacement therapy (ERT) is the administration of the hormone estrogen, usually together with progestin, to replace hormones no longer produced by the ovaries. Historically, ERT (also called hormone replacement therapy, or HRT) was given on a short-term basis to relieve the symptoms of menopause. The trend today, however, is to give long-term ERT for the purpose of preventing heart disease and osteoporosis, conditions that are increasingly likely to develop in women after menopause.

Estrogen therapy has the potential to reduce greatly a woman's risk of developing and dying from heart disease, particularly from coronary artery disease. A number of studies show that taking estrogen after menopause can decrease the incidence of certain risk factors associated with heart disease and can also substantially lower the death rate from heart attacks. One of the most commonly cited of these studies, the Nurses' Health Study, conducted by researchers at the Brigham and Women's Hospital and the Harvard Medical School in Boston, involved 48,470 postmenopausal nurses, who were followed for 10 years. Of these women, those who took estrogen had a heart attack rate almost half that of the women who took no replacement therapy.

A drawback to this and most of the other studies is that the women who were taking ERT may also have had a higher standard of living and been inclined to take better care of their health in general, factors that may have made them less vulnerable to heart attacks, with or without ERT. In an ideal study similar groups of women would be randomly selected to take, or not take, ERT and then would be compared years later to see which group had more heart attacks. In the Nurses' Study and similar research, women made their own choice about whether to take the drug, and this nonrandom factor may have skewed the results. The Women's Health Initiative, a large-scale government-sponsored study, aims, among other things, to determine just who will benefit from ERT and under what conditions, but data from that study will not be forthcoming until 2007.

▸ Weighing the risks and benefits

The growing consensus in the medical world is that estrogen therapy—continued for one or even two decades—prolongs life for most women, largely because the risk of developing and dying from heart disease is so high in women past 50. Lowering this risk even a bit, say advocates of ERT, can have huge repercussions in terms of saving lives and preserving the quality of life, despite the other risks.

After age 50 the risk of developing coronary artery disease is about 45 percent, and the risk of dying from heart disease is about 30 percent. In addition, the risk of incurring an osteoporosis-related fracture is 40 percent. Taking estrogen seems to decrease these risks substantially, and when it is combined with progestins (see below), ERT does not significantly increase the risk of endometrial cancer. In contrast, there is the possibility that ERT may increase the risk of developing breast cancer from about 10 percent to about 13 percent. As for gallstones, most clinicians feel that the slight increase associated with ERT has only negligible effects on a woman's overall health and longevity. All of this makes ERT sound quite appealing for the average woman.

But of course no one is average. Each individual has her own risk of developing heart disease or breast cancer, based on her own health and family history, as well as other risk factors. In addition, many of the judgments about the advisability of ERT are based on health risks for white women—and these may not apply to women of other races and backgrounds. Also, some women may find that they experience intolerable side effects when they use various forms of ERT.

For all of these reasons, each woman must consider her personal situation—not to mention her individual feelings about quality of life—and discuss these matters with her clinician before making a decision about ERT.

There are some women for whom ERT may simply be inappropriate. These include women who have had breast or uterine cancer or who currently have active liver disease. Women who have histories of stroke, heart attacks, and circulatory disorders involving blood clots have also traditionally been counseled against ERT, but many clinicians now feel that ERT is reasonable for these women so long as the problems were not related to high levels of estrogen (such as may have occurred during oral contraceptive use or pregnancy). For women who are at particularly high risk for coronary artery disease, such as smokers and women with hypertension or diabetes, the benefits of estrogen replacement far outweigh the risks. Replacement doses of estrogen apparently have little effect on blood pressure and seem to be safe even in women with mild hypertension. Nor does ERT appear to alter a woman's lifetime risk of stroke. Women with high levels of triglycerides in the blood or very high blood pressure should weigh the pros and cons carefully with their physicians. These women need closer monitoring after starting ERT to be sure it does not exacerbate the underlying condition.

There is evidence linking both estrogens and progestins to migraines, plus some circumstantial evidence indicating that these hormones probably have something to do with who gets headaches and when. Even so, while some women find that ERT exacerbates their headaches, just as many others find that it provides relief or no change at all. The best strategy is probably a little personal experimentation, with the understanding that if one hormone regimen makes migraines worse, it might be worth trying another one (such as a lower dose of estrogen or a transdermal patch) before abandoning the idea of ERT altogether.

Because the estrogen used for ERT is about 10 times less powerful than the estrogen used in oral contraceptives, the risks and benefits associated with birth control pills cannot necessarily be extended to ERT. In fact, several of the more serious risks and complications once associated with ERT were based on doses of estrogen much higher than are now generally prescribed. Daily doses of estrogen were once as high as 1.25 to 2.5 milligrams; today the standard dose is only 0.625 mg. Usually taken daily, this dosage seems to confer the same protective effects as higher doses which are more likely to overstimulate breast and uterine tissues.

Finally, whatever her personal risk factors, every woman who is using ERT should have an annual pelvic and breast examination. She should also have a mammogram done when therapy is initiated and then at yearly intervals thereafter. Women with a uterus who are on unopposed estrogens (for example, women who for whatever reason cannot tolerate the side effects of progestins) need to have yearly endometrial biopsies to check for cancerous or precancerous changes. These women may sometimes experience abnormal vaginal bleeding, including withdrawal bleeding (on the days

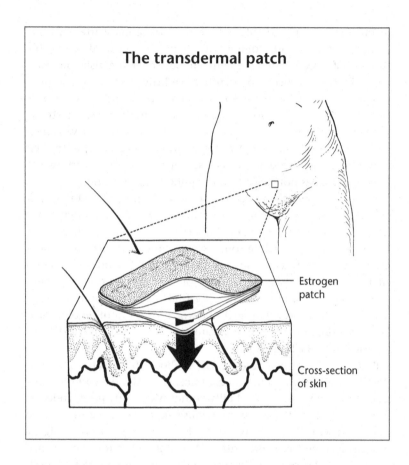

The transdermal patch

Estrogen patch

Cross-section of skin

when the estrogen is not taken) and irregular bleeding—which may but does not necessarily indicate an endometrial problem. Regular endometrial biopsies are generally unnecessary for women using combinations of estrogens and progestins unless they experience heavy, irregular, or prolonged bleeding (more than a normal menstrual period).

▸ How is ERT administered?
The most commonly prescribed ERT in the United States includes mixtures of several forms of estrogen taken from the urine of pregnant mares. Called conjugated estrogens, these preparations are sold

under trade names such as Premarin. Natural forms of estrogen (manufactured in the laboratory), which are less potent than conjugated estrogens, are also sometimes used—estradiol (Estrace and Estraderm), estropipate (Ogen), and esterified estrogens (Estratab).

Since the 1970s researchers have known that supplementary estrogen when taken by itself ("unopposed" estrogen) significantly increases the risk of endometrial cancer. This increased risk can be virtually eliminated, however, when estrogens are taken in combination with progestins. These are synthetic compounds that behave much like the hormone progesterone, and most of them have mild androgenic (virilizing) properties. In contrast to the progestins used in oral contraceptives—which tend to have the strongest virilizing properties—the most common form of progestin used in ERT, medroxyprogesterone acetate (Provera or Cycrin), is substantially less potent.

ERT can be administered in the form of pills or absorbed through the skin from transdermal patches (see illustration). Because hormones from patches (such as Estraderm) enter the bloodstream directly, they bypass the digestive system and are not immediately processed in the liver.

Pharmaceutical companies are scurrying to develop new formulations of estrogens and progestins, including skin creams and implants (some of which are already available in Europe), which they hope will prove to be safer than current options but just as beneficial.

Exercise

In the nineteenth century, many doctors warned that strenuous physical activity would destroy a woman's femininity and reproductive capacity. Today we know that regular exercise and physical fitness are important in preventing coronary artery disease and diabetes, in relieving stress, and in controlling weight gain and hypertension.

When it comes to protecting the heart, exercise that significantly increases the heart rate and the body's demand for oxygen is believed to decrease the risk of coronary artery disease and high blood pressure by strengthening the heart and lungs, widening the blood vessels, improving the efficiency with which oxygen is delivered to body tissues, and boosting levels of high-density lipoprotein. Examples of aerobic exercise include jogging, brisk walking, long-distance or uphill bicycling, swimming, and dancing.

There are many different ways to incorporate aerobic or any other exercise into one's weekly routine. Specific routines may vary according to a woman's individual capacity, lifestyle, and interests as well as her stage of life and overall health. Women should not forget to take into account the amount of exercise they get as part of daily life. A woman whose job involves a great deal of walking or manual labor—or a young mother who spends half her day running up and down the stairs, vacuuming floors, and chasing after toddlers—will obviously have different supplementary exercise needs than a woman who drives to work, sits all day at a desk, and pays someone to clean her house.

All women just beginning an exercise routine should start slowly and only gradually increase the frequency and length of sessions. Most physiologists recommend that women aim to reach about 75 to 85 percent of the average maximum heart rate for their age group during aerobic exercise. This rate can be calculated by subtracting the woman's age from 220. Thus, a 40-year-old woman has an average maximum heart rate of 180 (220 minus 40) beats per minute, and at peak condition her heart rate should equal 75 percent of that, or 135 beats per minute. Beginning exercisers should be satisfied reaching just 50 to 60 percent of their average maximum heart rate during workouts.

Among adolescents and healthy premenopausal women, most exercise physiologists recommend that some form of continuous aerobic exercises be performed 3 to 5 times a week for at least 20 minutes at a stretch. These should be preceded by about 5 minutes of warmup flexibility exercises and followed by 5 or 10 minutes of cool-down exercises—such as deep breathing, walking, or stretching. There is no harm in doing aerobic exercises on a daily basis, though benefits from such diligence seem no greater than those from a 3 to 5 day a week routine.

Pregnant women who previously engaged in swimming, jogging, tennis, dancing, or brisk walking can usually continue these activities, so long as they make sure to keep their pulse rate under 140 beats per minute (well-trained athletes may be able to go a little higher). Even women who have led sedentary lives before pregnancy generally find that a regular exercise program during pregnancy decreases fatigue and helps improve muscle tone and endurance, thus easing the physical stress of both pregnancy and childbirth. Regular exercise during pregnancy can also help prevent excess weight gain and make it easier to shed pounds afterward. Information about exercise during pregnancy is available from clinicians as well as from almost any pregnancy book. In addition, local YWCAs, hospitals, and park districts often offer exercise classes designed specifically for pregnant and postpartum women.

Among middle-aged women, new studies indicate that a regular aerobic routine can significantly decrease the risks of coronary artery disease and noninsulin-dependent diabetes. The benefits of exercise continue into the 70s, 80s, and beyond.

Finally, increasing one's physical activity plays a major role in any successful weight loss program (see Weight Control).

▸ What are the risks and complications of aerobic exercise?

When exercise produces dizziness, sharp pain, pressure in the chest, or shortness of breath, it should be stopped immediately. If symptoms continue, a clinician should be consulted.

Before beginning any active exercise program, a woman who has been sedentary should have a thorough physical examination. This is especially important for women over 45 and for those who have heart disease, diabetes, or hypertension.

Quitting Smoking

In general, a middle-aged woman who smokes is 3 times more likely to die of coronary artery disease and 5 times more likely to die of a stroke than a nonsmoking woman of the same age. Women smokers over the age of 35 who use birth control pills have an increased risk of both heart attack and stroke. Even women who smoke as few as 1 to 4 cigarettes per day have a higher risk of cardiovascular death than nonsmoking women. Contrary to common belief, reduced tar and nicotine cigarettes do not seem to afford any protection against these risks. No level of tobacco use is known to be safe.

Cigarette smoking is the leading preventable cause of death for both men and women in the United States. It has been blamed for an estimated 419,000 deaths per year in this country (or 1 in every 5 deaths) from cardiovascular disease, stroke, and cancers of the lung, mouth, larynx, esophagus (windpipe), bladder, pancreas, and stomach. Smokers have higher rates of peptic ulcer disease, are more susceptible to upper respiratory infections, and have more cataracts than nonsmokers.

Most of what we know about the ill effects of smoking is based on large-scale studies in men. But the evidence is becoming increasingly clear that a woman who smokes like a man can expect to get sick and die like a man.

▸ What are the benefits of quitting?
Many of the risks associated with cigarette smoking can be reversed or substantially reduced by quitting. An ex-smoker's excess risk of dying from cardiovascular disease, for example, is eliminated in the first year after quitting. Ten to 15 years after stopping, an ex-smoker's overall risk of death is close to that of a person who has never smoked. This is true no matter how old a woman is or how long or heavily she has smoked. It is even true for women who stop smoking after they have developed some smoking-related symptom—although the more damage that has been done, the longer it will take to reverse it.

The biggest gains come to smokers who quit when they are young, when they have been exposed to relatively few cigarettes, and when they are still free of smoking-related disease. The health hazards associated with the small amount of weight that many women gain after stopping smoking are minuscule compared with the hazards associated with smoking.

▸ What is the best way to quit?

For the most part, awareness of health risks is not enough to motivate people to quit. Over 90 percent of current smokers know full well that smoking is harmful to their health, and yet a vague fear of some future disease is not enough to keep them from smoking. What does seem to motivate many smokers to quit, however, is the development of a smoking-related symptom such as chest pain, a persistent cough, or breathlessness in the smoker herself or in a close family member or friend. These symptoms may or may not be related to the cigarette smoking, but they often scare a smoker into seeing herself as personally vulnerable. Social pressure also plays a role in evoking the desire to quit.

Most smokers today say they would like to stop and have made at least one concerted attempt to do so. It often takes two or three serious efforts before this mission is accomplished. This is because quitting is more than a matter of willpower. Smoking cessation is often a learning process in which mistakes made in the first attempt help improve the odds of success in the next one. In fact, most smokers go through a slow series of psychological stages before they are able to stop smoking. The first is characterized by an initial lack of interest in quitting. Next the smoker begins to think about the health risks associated with cigarettes and contemplates quitting—someday. Eventually something—whether the development of a symptom or pressure from peers or health professionals—will stimulate active plans to quit within the next month. At last the actual "quitting day" arrives, and the person stops smoking. The final stage arrives when the nonsmoking is maintained permanently.

One thing that makes quitting difficult is that many smokers are both physically and psychologically dependent on cigarettes. When smoking is abandoned, withdrawal symptoms may make life difficult. Symptoms of nicotine withdrawal include ▸ cravings for a cigarette; ▸ irritability, anxiety, impatience, and anger; ▸ difficulty concentrating; ▸ excessive hunger; and ▸ sleep disturbances. These symptoms usually start within a few hours of the last cigarette. They are strongest during the first 2 to 3 days of abstinence but gradually diminish over 2 to 3 weeks. Just how severe these symptoms are depends on the smoker's prior level of nicotine intake. Since most of these symptoms (except the craving for cigarettes) are not specifically related to smoking, many people do not recognize them for what they are.

Despite some evidence that nicotine withdrawal symptoms are more severe during the luteal phase (the second half) of a woman's menstrual cycle, quitting earlier in the cycle does not seem to improve the chances of success. A better solution to overcoming nicotine withdrawal symptoms involves behavioral methods. These methods help smokers identify cues to smoking and let them break the link between the trigger and the behavior and learn how to handle urges to smoke. Such skills can be learned at home from booklets or videotapes or in a formal group program. If necessary, a doctor may also prescribe nicotine gum or skin patches to ease the transition from smoking to nonsmoking.

Anyone trying to quit smoking should be aware of the insidious effects of coffee and alcohol—drugs that are more commonly used by smokers than nonsmokers. Many clinicians advise ex-smokers to avoid alcohol temporarily after quitting, since drinking alcoholic beverages seems to induce relapses in cigarette smoking. As for coffee, smoking tends to increase the rate at which caffeine is excreted from the body. When cigarettes are abandoned, therefore, the amount of caffeine left in the blood after the standard dose of coffee is higher than before, and the result is unaccustomed jitteriness.

Because smokers use cigarettes to relax or relieve negative emotions such as anger, anxiety, and frustration, quitting often makes it difficult to get through their daily routine. Losing this coping tool may be particularly difficult for women, many of whom find it hard to express anger directly. Abandoning cigarettes can also be difficult for the many smokers conditioned to light up a cigarette whenever they wake up in the morning or whenever they have a cup of coffee. Despite the best of intentions in the person trying to quit, these activities trigger the desire for a cigarette the way the ringing of a bell triggered Pavlov's dog to salivate. Again, behavioral modification strategies are often the best way to circumvent these psychological and behavioral barriers to quitting.

Another reason why so many smokers continue to use cigarettes is that they have a certain ambivalence about abandoning the habit. This is particularly true of women smokers. Although women are about as likely as men to quit smoking successfully, there are certain issues that complicate the process for them. Chief among these is concern about weight. The truth is that smokers who quit do wind up weighing on average 5 to 10 pounds more than people of comparable age and height who never smoked. This is probably because the metabolic rate decreases when nicotine is withdrawn, although it may also have something to do with a tendency among ex-smokers to substitute food for cigarettes. Whatever the explanation, approximately 4 out of 5 smokers do gain weight after abandoning cigarettes, and women who quit smoking seem to gain more weight than men. Given the cultural pressure on women to be slender, this fact certainly discourages many women smokers from abandoning the habit.

Nonetheless, given all the risks of smoking, the best approach might be a change in attitude about a few excess pounds. After all, in the grand scheme of things, 5 to 10 pounds of excess weight does not represent a serious health risk. Only about 1 in 10 women ex-smokers gains more than 25 pounds, although heavier smokers (more than 25 cigarettes per day) do gain somewhat more weight than lighter smokers. In most cases a woman should expect only a small increase in weight, which can be shed—if she wishes—once the attempt to stop smoking has been accomplished. Using nicotine gum may also delay weight gain—at least until the gum use stops. Avoiding high-calorie snacks and increasing physical activity can also help. But trying to diet and give up cigarettes at the same time is almost always counterproductive on both counts.

Another obstacle to quitting is the frequent lack of social support. The evidence is abundantly clear, for example, that smokers whose efforts are bolstered by partners, family, and friends are more likely to succeed than smokers without such support. Moreover, smokers with a nonsmoking spouse are more likely to quit than smokers with spouses who smoke. And yet women smokers are less likely than men smokers to have spouses or partners who actively support their effort to quit. For these reasons, women trying to give up cigarettes have to find ways to ask family and friends to restrict smoking to outdoor areas or to limited areas in order to ensure a smoke-free area in the home or workplace. Sometimes it can also help to seek additional social support in a formal smoking cessation program.

A final obstacle to quitting that plagues women in particular involves mood disorders—especially depression. It now appears that smokers have more symptoms of depression and histories of major depression than nonsmokers. Some researchers also suspect that quitting may actually precipitate depression in smokers who have a history of major depression, and that resuming smoking may elevate mood. Also, depressed smokers are less likely to stop smoking than smokers who are not depressed. Since depression is about 3 times as common in women as in men, all of these observations are particularly relevant to women who smoke. It is important to have symptoms of depression treated before one attempts to stop smoking. In addition, any woman who is trying to stop smoking should watch out for symptoms of depression.

In all cases, anyone trying to quit smoking should not be discouraged by temporary setbacks. If going "cold turkey" is too difficult, it may help to start by gradually cutting down or switching to cigarettes low in tar and nicotine. If quitting alone is impossible, a woman can join a formal nonsmoking program or support group or enlist the help of a clinician. Contacting a local chapter of the American Lung Association or the American Cancer Society (listed in the phone book) is another good way to find helpful smoking cessation programs and other information. Many of these programs not only offer intensive training in behavioral techniques but also offer social support from a counselor and other group members, and this may be particularly valuable to women who smoke.

▸ Does nicotine replacement therapy work?

Giving up cigarettes involves two separate challenges: the addiction to nicotine has to be overcome, and the habit of smoking cigarettes has to be broken. Nicotine replacement therapy—in the form of either nicotine gum or nicotine patches—can help separate these two challenges by allowing the smoker to focus on breaking the smoking habit before dealing with the nicotine addiction. Although many smokers are able to overcome the addiction on their own, nicotine gum or patches may be helpful for people who experience severe nicotine withdrawal symptoms.

Both nicotine gum and nicotine patches can be quite safe and effective—even in smokers with coronary artery disease—if used properly. They work even better if used in conjunction with a behavioral counseling program that teaches the smoker how to break the cigarette habit. Both of these forms of nicotine therapy work by replacing nicotine in amounts just large enough to block the symptoms of nicotine withdrawal but too small to reproduce the pleasure of smoking. In contrast to smoking, which leads to fluctuating levels of nicotine in the bloodstream, both the gum and the patch produce relatively constant blood levels of nicotine.

Women who have recently had a heart attack or who have unstable angina or serious arrhythmias should not use either form of nicotine replacement, nor should women who continue to smoke cigarettes. Researchers still do not know if either product is safe for use during pregnancy.

Nicotine patches. A nicotine patch is applied to a hairless spot on the upper arm or torso on the first morning that the smoker plans to quit. It contains a fixed amount of nicotine which is released in fixed doses and absorbed through the skin throughout the day. Three of the four brands of patches now on the market are worn for 24 hours and replaced the next morning; the fourth product is removed before bedtime so that there is a patch-free period. Most patches need to be used for about 2 to 3 months, during which time the dose of nicotine contained in them can be gradually tapered off.

Local skin irritation is the most common side effect of the nicotine patch, but this can usually be treated with topical steroid preparations. The patch is inappropriate for women with widespread skin eruptions. Occasionally people using the patches find they have vivid dreams, insomnia, and nervousness. To control these side effects, it often helps to remove the patch at bedtime or reduce the dose of nicotine in the patch.

Nicotine gum. Nicotine gum is somewhat more difficult to use correctly. Available in two different strengths, it is not supposed to be chewed like regular gum. Instead, each piece should be chewed only long enough to release the nicotine, which produces a peppery flavor, and then the gum should be parked between the cheek and gum for a few minutes, or until the peppery taste or tingling has disappeared. At this point the gum should be chewed a few more times until the nicotine is released, and then parked between the cheek and gum once again. This entire process should be repeated for about half an hour or until no more peppery taste is released. It is important not to drink any liquid while the gum is in the mouth and to avoid drinking any acidic beverages such as coffee for at least an hour or two before using the gum.

Most people need to chew between 9 and 12 pieces of gum a day (it helps to try chewing one piece every hour) to prevent withdrawal symptoms, although some heavy smokers may need as many as 30 pieces. After 6 weeks of use, the number of pieces can be gradually reduced.

Nicotine gum use often produces a number of minor side effects. Many of these—such as nausea, dyspepsia, hiccups, and dizziness—are related to nicotine withdrawal. Others are related to chewing, and include sore jaw and mouth ulcers. About 5 to 10 percent of nicotine gum users develop a long-term dependence on the gum.

Nicotine gum should not be used by women with temporomandibular joint syndrom, a common disorder of the joint that connects the jawbone to the skull.

▸What other medical treatments are available?

The FDA has just approved an antidepressant, bupropion (Wellbutrin), as an aid in smoking cessation. Evidence shows that smokers attempting to quit have a higher success rate when they take this drug, as compared with those who use conventional techniques without any drug treatment.

Bupropion is not chemically related to other classes of antidepressants, which include selective serotonin reuptake inhibitors and tricyclic antidepressants. The exact mechanism for bupropion's action is not known. It is known, however, that smokers with a history of depression have a fair chance of experiencing a depressive episode after quitting. People with persistent nicotine withdrawal symptoms after quitting are also more likely to experience depression. Since women are more vulnerable to depression than men, may become physiologically addicted to nicotine more readily, and may experience more serious withdrawal symptoms, bupropion may be particularly helpful for women who are trying to quit smoking.

Stress Reduction

According to highly popularized reports some years back, people tagged as having the infamous high-stress "Type A" personality—characterized by high levels of competitiveness, ambition, hostility, impatience, abruptness, and obsessiveness—were particularly susceptible to heart disease. Although newer studies indicate that at least some people with such personality types may thrive (particularly if they are successful), many doctors still feel that chronic troubling emotions, interpersonal conflicts, and depression—as well as plain old stress and anxiety—may indeed be risk factors in heart disease.

Several animal experiments and clinical observations of humans have suggested some plausible physiological mechanisms that help explain why and how emotions and behaviors can affect the heart. For example, even minimal stimuli such as casual conversation can provoke acute elevations in blood pressure. Blood pressure will rise even more—and for a longer time—when emotions such as anger or fear are aroused. Anxiety seems to evoke the greatest increase in women's blood pressure, whereas anger evokes the greatest rise in men's. According to some researchers, such brief elevations, occurring many thousands of times, may damage vulnerable blood vessel walls (see High Blood Pressure).

Furthermore, mammals under stress show physiological changes that encourage blood clotting (to protect the animal against blood loss from a potential injury) and increase blood flow to vital organs and to muscles necessary for fighting or fleeing. Increased blood clotting and greater demands placed on the heart caused by these changes can set the stage for a heart attack. Other studies show that emotional changes can influence the autonomic nervous system, which in turn regulates the heart's rate and rhythm. Sustained stress may lead people to overeat, smoke more, or neglect exercise, and these poor health habits impact badly on the heart.

Of course, none of this necessarily means that people with Type A personalities should try to transform themselves into the calmer, less ambitious Type Bs. So far there is no convincing evidence that changing emotional responses can actually prevent heart disease or other serious disorders, and "personality" may be almost impossible to change anyway. And given that Type A behavior often leads to great rewards in our society, trying to change it may provoke even greater anxiety in many people.

A person already at risk for heart disease may, nevertheless, want to think about ways she can change her behavior or attitude so as to reduce the frustration, stress, and anxiety in her life, especially if doing so will result in a more enjoyable life. More important, anyone experiencing considerable stress would be wise to pay special attention to eliminating other habits or conditions more closely linked to disease—such as smoking or high blood pressure.

▸ Who is likely to develop high levels of stress?

The modern woman is said to be drowning in a sea of stress. In addition to the traditional sources of stress—such as the demands of young children and aging parents—many women today also face considerable stress in the workplace. Since the late 1960s, 300 hours of work—including time spent at work as well as time spent caring for a household—have been added to a working woman's annual schedule. "Working moms" are the major breadwinner in many two-parent families, and the only breadwinner in the vast majority of single-parent families. Although both men and women often feel stressed from repetitive, unstimulating work, stress for women is compounded by pay inequity (women's pay is still on average only 71 percent that of men with comparable training and responsibilities), the lack of adequate health insurance and other benefits (especially in parts of the service sector where the majority of women work), a "glass ceiling" and "mommy track" that prevent women from rising to positions of authority as often or as rapidly as men with comparable abilities, and, above all else, the difficulty of balancing work and family responsibilities.

A report by the U.S. Department of Labor has revealed that working women rank stress as their greatest everyday problem. The largest number of complaints came from women in their 40s who had professional and managerial jobs, and from single mothers who said that their biggest problem is balancing family and work, including finding affordable childcare.

Interpersonal conflict seems to be particularly stressful to women, whereas competition and intellectual challenge are more stressful to men. Studies have shown that competitive challenges lead to greater than average elevations in blood pressure—even during sleep—in men with Type A personalities. Such findings suggest that difficult work permanently damages the circulatory system (or, alternatively, that men with Type A personalities or high blood pressure tend to choose high-pressure jobs). But when it comes to women, the pressures of work seem much less likely to affect blood pressure. The only exceptions are women in top management jobs.

What does seem to send women's blood pressure soaring are interpersonal conflicts and strains at home, especially problems with partners and children. These findings make things look particularly bleak for young women in upper management who go home to children and other family responsibilities. Men tend to relax after leaving a high-pressure job, but women with equivalent jobs often get no relief. This unremitting stress of the "second shift" is what ultimately sends many women around the bend, emotionally and, eventually, physically.

During their reproductive years, these young women may have a built-in buffer against the physical effects of stress because of the protective effects of estrogen—particularly its effect on serum cholesterol levels. In one study, for example, even Type A women had serum cholesterol levels similar to those of less competitive (and less stressed) women and much lower than those of Type A men. Although LDL cholesterol levels (which have been linked to heart attack risk) were higher in women managers, protective HDL levels also remained high in all women, regardless of the nature of their job or their personality type.

▸ How can women alleviate stress?

Some women may handle the stress in their lives better than men because they are better able to identify and deal with it. By venting their frustrations with friends or even allowing themselves a good cry, women may be dispelling some of the most toxic effects of

Stress-reducing techniques

Change your environment

Reduce external stress such as noise and pollution
Reduce stimulation at home when possible
Reduce stimulation at work when possible
Reduce threats to your physical safety

Change your behavior

Eat a balanced diet
Get enough sleep
Get adequate exercise
Learn relaxation techniques or meditation
Cut back on alcohol and caffeine consumption
Reduce exposure to situations that involve conflict
Take a time-management course
Undergo hypnosis

Develop a new attitude

Set limits for yourself and others
Become more aware of other options
Become more aware of what you are feeling
Be more willing to express what you are feeling
Become more confident about your own perceptions
Become more aware of the possibility of internal change

stress. Aware that their lives are stressful, women may purposefully adopt a healthier lifestyle, perhaps choosing foods more carefully, losing weight, cutting out cigarettes, getting enough sleep, or embarking on an exercise plan—which often helps vent frustration in and of itself.

Women who feel overwhelmed by stress may want to try adopting some of these stress-resistant strategies (see chart). Delineating specific sources of stress, prioritizing demands, and learning to find satisfaction in less frustrating areas of life can work wonders. Establishing a stable daily routine, actively seeking social support, and believing in one's personal ability to solve problems can help some women better manage stress. For extremely compulsive women, stress can be reduced by accepting the necessity, sometimes, of a temporary disruption in one's daily routine, or realizing that one cannot solve all of one's problems at the same time.

Relaxation exercises can often undo some of the stresses of everyday life. Transcendental meditation and yoga, practiced over many months or years, have been credited with lowering elevated blood pressure and with making people feel less anxious and out of control, as has hypnosis. In some situations becoming more assertive can alleviate stress: it may be helpful to speak up about job frustrations, or to investigate a company's grievance procedures. Taking a course in time management or in meditation techniques has given many women relief during periods of unusual stress.

Weight Control

The burning questions among weight researchers today seem to be: ▸ What range of weights for a given height is consistent with good health among adults? ▸ And do these ranges change with age? That is, is some modest weight gain during adulthood consistent with good health?

According to the 1990 *Report of the Dietary Guidelines Advisory Committee* (issued by the U.S. Department of Agriculture and the Department of Health and Human Services) and analysis done at the National Institute of Aging's Gerontology Research Center, some weight gain after age 35 is consistent with good health in both men and women. That is, based on actuarial tables from life insurance companies, they conclude that mortality rates overall are lowest among people who gain a few pounds per decade of adulthood. The *Guidelines* do not differentiate between the weights of men and women, which implies that women, whose bones and muscles weigh less than men's, can have a higher relative percentage of fat than men of the same height and still be considered healthy (see chart).

But a study of over 115,000 nurses by Harvard University researchers has recently thrown some cold water on these rosy recommendations. It showed that the risk of coronary artery disease is greater for women at the high end of the "normal" range as defined by the USDA *Guidelines* and lower for women who are below the low end of the "normal" range. Women of average weight had about a 50 percent higher risk of heart attack than women who were 15 percent less than average weight. And even for women within the normal range, modest weight gain after age 18 was associated with an increased risk of heart disease. Women who gained 10 pounds or less in early to middle adulthood had the lowest risk of heart attacks. The authors of this study recommend going back to the 1959 Metropolitan Life tables for "ideal weights," which make no allowances for age and recommend lower weights for women of any age (see chart on page 120; the 1983 Met Life weights are also given for comparison).

USDA suggested weights		
Height without shoes	Weight without clothes	
	19 to 34 years	Over 35 years
5'0"	97–128	108–138
5'1"	101–132	111–143
5'2"	104–137	115–148
5'3"	107–141	119–152
5'4"	111–146	122–157
5'5"	114–150	126–162
5'6"	118–155	130–167
5'7"	121–160	134–172
5'8"	125–164	138–178
5'9"	129–169	142–183
5'10"	132–174	146–188
5'11"	136–179	151–194
6'0"	140–184	155–199

One of the sticking points seems to be whether one looks at overall mortality (as the USDA *Guidelines* do) or at heart disease, which is the greatest cause of death among women after middle age. Modest weight gain seems to be associated with a lower overall risk of dying, but also seems to raise the chances that one will die of a heart attack. Do slightly heavier people have a lower incidence of cancer and other life-threatening conditions that offsets their risk of heart disease? Perhaps, but the data are equivocal at best.

There are two things that we do know for sure: ▸ Those who gain a considerable amount of weight while passing through the adult years die at an earlier than average age. ▸ And though Americans have been getting somewhat heavier over the last few decades, their life expectancy has continued to increase, which suggests that a few extra pounds are not a grave threat to health overall.

Comparison of 1959 and 1983 Metropolitan height and weight tables

Height without shoes	Weight without clothing	
	1959	1983
4'10"	92–121	100–131
4'11"	95–124	101–134
5'0"	98–127	103–137
5'1"	101–130	105–140
5'2"	104–134	108–144
5'3"	107–138	111–148
5'4"	110–142	114–152
5'5"	114–146	117–156
5'6"	118–150	120–160
5'7"	122–154	123–164
5'8"	126–159	126–167
5'9"	130–164	129–170
5'10"	134–169	132–173

Note on 1959 table: For women 18–25 years, subtract one pound for each year under 25.

▸ What is the best plan for weight loss?

There is now good evidence that the greatest health benefits from weight loss occur with the first 10 to 20 percent of excess body fat that is lost—which is the easiest weight to lose. Setting realistic goals usually means aiming to lose no more than 10 percent of body weight. Thus, a 160-pound woman should aim to lose no more than 16 pounds. Then, if necessary, a new goal of another 10 percent can be set after the new weight has been maintained for a year. This 10 percent reduction in body weight will reduce the woman's risk for coronary artery disease, diabetes, and hypertension while still leaving her with a normal (not overly slowed) metabolic rate. Unless a woman weighs 20 percent more than the healthy ideal for her height, increasing exercise and activity levels and developing healthy eating habits usually makes more sense over the long run than weight loss diets per se.

In general, any valid weight control plan will emphasize gradual weight loss (a pound a week). Crash dieting or starvation, while often producing a gratifying weight (or, more accurately, water) drop over the first few days, only lowers metabolic rate, which ultimately makes it harder to burn fat. Fasts and unbalanced diets often result in the loss of lean tissue and important nutrients. Over-the-counter liquid protein diets, supplemented with vitamins and minerals, are much safer, but they rarely produce long-term weight loss.

Because it takes about 3,500 calories to produce a single pound of fat, losing 20 pounds requires restricting caloric intake over time by a total of $20 \times 3,500 = 70,000$ calories. But calorie cutting alone does not ensure a safe or successful diet. Any safe and effective diet plan for an adult woman should emphasize starches, fruits, and vegetables, and include low-fat or nonfat milk and yogurt to meet calcium needs. Intake of simple sugars and fats should be limited. Such a plan will call for eating several meals and snacks distributed throughout the day, a daily caloric consumption of at least 1,000 to 1,200 calories, adequate protein, and a fat intake limited to 20 percent of total calories. In a 1,200 to 1,500 calorie a day plan, this means eating no more than 27 to 33 grams of fat a day. In a 1,800 calorie diet, it means eating no more than 44 grams of fat. An easy way to estimate and keep track of fat intake is to use a fat gram counter book, read food labels, and record total fat intake in a food diary.

Increasing one's physical activity plays a major role in any successful weight loss program. Exercise sessions that last longer than 30 minutes are particularly helpful, since after this length of time the body starts burning body fat (in addition to carbohydrate sugars) for energy. Some studies show that exercising soon after a meal can boost the metabolic rate even more than exercise in general and thus also boost the number of calories burned.

Whatever the plan, women tend to lose less weight than men do because they have a lower lean body mass. People who are less overweight to begin with, or older, also tend to lose weight with more difficulty.

Many women find group programs such as Weight Watchers helpful. These organizations provide education and diet advice, as well as peer support and encouragement. The best programs focus on making lifetime changes in nutritious food choices and exercise patterns, as well as reversing destructive attitudes about food and eating. They also rarely involve buying expensive "substitute" foods and vitamins. Often these groups offer behavior modification programs that can be helpful in changing abnormal eating patterns.

▸ Weight loss drugs

Although some researchers believe that there is clear and convincing evidence that modern appetite suppressant drugs (such as fenfluramine and phentermine) are effective and safe, others argue that most people who try them lose only a small amount of weight, which is soon regained. They also argue that drugs can too easily become a substitute for education, exercise, and good nutrition, so ultimately maintaining the new weight becomes difficult. In addition, appetite suppressants can cause annoying side effects such as dry mouth and drowsiness as well as rare but life-treatening complications (see Obesity). All in all, these drugs are no substitute for good nutrition, healthy eating habits, and exercise. They may be of benefit to people with a long history of losing weight and regaining it—especially if they already have complications of obesity.

Some patients find that hypnosis, acupuncture, and other alternative therapies help them control their appetite and change their eating habits. To date, scientific investigation of the safety and effectiveness of most of these approaches has not been undertaken.

▸ What are the risks and complications of dieting?

Despite the health risks inherent in obesity, the very act of dieting can be risky for some women. Not only have decreased self-esteem and self-confidence been associated with chronic dieting, but also the desire for thinness, particularly in women, has been associated with a high prevalence of eating disorders such as anorexia nervosa, bulimia nervosa, and "binge eating disorder." Adult women dieters who have little weight to lose (less than 10 percent of their weight) may end up losing excessive lean body mass rather than unwanted fat.

On the plus side, it no longer appears that yo-yo dieting—cyclic weight loss and gain—poses any particular risks to health. Earlier and widely publicized reports of this belief were based on studies that failed to differentiate between people who lost weight voluntarily and those who lost it owing to illness.

Dieting can be particularly unwise in adolescence, a time of critical growth and development. Not only can caloric deprivation interfere with physical growth, but also an obsession with thinness and dieting can result in eating disorders or a lifetime of poor self-image. Increasing activity and making healthy food choices make much more sense for the mildly overweight adolescent. Although dieting may be appropriate in the case of a severe weight problem, this should be initiated only under the guidance of a clinician. As with all eating disorders, family therapy may be advisable in some cases as well.

▸ What health factors should be considered along with weight?

An individual woman should not assume she is unhealthy just because the scale registers a few pounds above or below the listed values. Weight is only one of a number of factors that help indicate a person's well-being. To evaluate overall health more meaningfully, the number on the scale must be considered along with physical fitness, family history, lifestyle factors such as cigarette smoking and alcohol use, and current medical and psychological health.

Evidence is accumulating that weight may not be as important in predicting heart disease as the ratio of fat to muscle. And whatever their weight, people who have large accumulations of fat around the abdomen have a risk of cardiovascular disease and diabetes far greater than that of people with large accumulations of fat around the hips or thighs. Also, fat itself may not be the issue, so much as cardiovascular fitness; a woman who exercises regularly but is still overweight may not need to worry about her heart's health. The

Harvard Nurses' Study showed that cigarette smoking (which is more prevalent among lean women) is a greater risk factor for heart disease than is body weight; and while women who have more than 2 alcoholic drinks per day are at risk for many life-threatening diseases, including alcoholism, women who drink more moderately (1 to 2 drinks per day) have a lower risk of heart disease than women who do not drink at all. And finally, estrogen replacement therapy (ERT) is known to reduce substantially the risk of heart disease in all women.

From some future study or reanalysis we may learn that an active woman who takes ERT, does not smoke, enjoys a glass of wine with dinner, and picks up a few pounds over the years has the best chance of living a long and healthy life. But until that definitive study is published, the jury is still out on the ideal weight for a healthy heart.

For More Information

The following resources are not intended to be exhaustive but to indicate possible starting points for any woman seeking more information on a given topic than this *Guide* provides. Most entries cite one or two books with up-to-date information and, when available, the names and addresses of organizations that provide reliable information and patient support. When appropriate, other resources, such as audiotapes, videotapes, and Internet sites and newsgroups, are listed.

Where to Look. Organizations usually are listed once, under the most inclusive entry.

Books. Most titles cited are in print and available through booksellers. The exceptions should be in the collections of most libraries.

Organizations. Addresses may have changed since the book went to press. The initial "1" has been dropped from all telephone numbers, since most areas of the country now have to dial 1 before long-distance calls.

Electronic resources. Resources are listed for the Internet and World Wide Web only. Also worth exploring are information and support groups available through commercial online services, such as America Online, CompuServe, and Prodigy. Accessing information on the World Wide Web requires an Internet connection and browser software, such as Netscape or Mosaic. Most Web addresses carry the standard prefix *http://*. Subscriptions to mailing lists also require e-mail capability, either through a direct Internet connection or a commercial online service. Readers who would like a general introduction to finding resources on the Internet can consult:

Daniel P. Dern, *The Internet Guide for New Users* (New York: McGraw-Hill, 1994).

General Resources

National Women's Health Resource Center
Suite 325
2440 M St. N.W.
Washington, DC 20037
202-293-6045
Publication: Bimonthly health update

National Black Women's Health Project (NBWHP)
1237 Ralph David Abernathy Blvd., S.W.
Atlanta, GA 30310
800-ASK-BWHP (800-275-2947)

National Institute on Aging
P.O. Box 8057
Gaithersburg, MD 20898-8057
800-222-2225

National Latina Health Organization (NLHO)
P.O. Box 7567
Oakland, CA 94601
510-534-1362

National Women's Health Network (NWHN)
514 10th Street NW
Washington DC 20004
202-347-1140

Native American Women's Health Education Resource Center
P.O. Box 572
Lake Andes, SD 57356
605-487-7072
Fax: 605-487-7964

Women of All Red Nations (WARN)
4511 N. Hermitage
Chicago IL 60640

Women of Color Partnership Program
Religious Coalition for Abortion Rights
1025 Vermont NW
Suite 1130
Washington, DC 20005
202-628-7700
Publication: *Common Ground, Different Planes,* newsletter on reproductive health issues for women of color.

OAM Public Information Center
Office of Alternative Medicine
National Institutes of Health
Suite 450
6120 Executive Blvd.
Rockville, MD 20892-9904
301-402-2466
General information packet available by return fax or mail by calling the main number.

Harvard Women's Health Watch
Harvard Medical School Health Publications Group
164 Longwood Avenue
Boston, Massachusetts 02115-5818
617-432-1485
A monthly newsletter that explores health topics unique to women.

Harvard Heart Letter
Harvard Medical School Health Publications Group
164 Longwood Avenue
Boston, MA 02115-5818
617-432-1485
A monthly newsletter featuring review articles and guidance on cardiovascular issues.

Women's Health Forum
6113 Abbey Road
Aptos, California 95003
408-662-8500
Fax: 408-662-1826
An interdisciplinary newsletter on health topics of interest to women.

The Black Women's Health Book: Speaking for Ourselves (Seattle: Seal Press, 1994).

Edward B. Diethrich and Carol Cohan, *Women and Heart Disease: What You Can Do to Stop the Number-One Killer of American Women* (New York: Ballantine, 1994).

Bill Moyers, *Healing and the Mind* (New York: Doubleday, 1993).

Frederic J. Pashkow and Charlotte Libov, *The Women's Heart Book: The Complete Guide to Keeping Your Heart Healthy and What to Do If Things Go Wrong* (New York: Dutton, 1993).

Coronary Artery Disease

American Heart Association
7272 Greenville Ave.
Dallas, TX 75231
214-373-6300
Publications: Two free pamphlets, "Fact Sheet on Heart Attack, Stroke, and Risk Factors" and "Why Risk Heart Attack? Seven Ways to Guard Your Heart."

Marianne J. Legato, *The Female Heart: The Truth about Women and Coronary Artery Disease* (New York: Avon, 1993).

Heart Failure

Marc A. Silver, *Success with Heart Failure: Help and Hope for Those with Congestive Heart Failure* (Washington, DC: Insight Books, 1994).

Diabetes

American Diabetes Association, Inc.
1660 Duke St.
Alexandria, VA 22314-3427
703-549-1500
800-ADA-DISC (800-232-3472)
Publication: *Diabetes and Pregnancy: What to Expect.*

Richard S. Beaser et al., *The Joslin Guide to Diabetes: A Program for Managing Your Treatment* (New York: Fireside, 1995).

Lester Henry, *The Black Health Library Guide to Diabetes* (New York: Henry Holt, 1993).

Lois Jovanovic-Peterson et al., *The Diabetic Woman: All Your Questions Answered* (New York: Tarcher, 1988).

High Cholesterol

National Heart, Lung, and Blood Institute
9000 Rockville Pike
Bethesda, MD 20892
301-496-4236
Publications: Free fact sheets on blood cholesterol (NIH publication 85-2696) and hyperlipoproteinemia (NIH publication 81-734).

American Heart Association
7272 Greenville Avenue
Dallas, Texas 75231
214-373-6300
(check phone book for local chapter)
Publications: "Nutrition Labeling: Food Selection Hints for Fat-Controlled Meals" and "Recipes for Fat-Controlled Low Cholesterol Meals from the American Heart Association Cookbook." Single copy free.

Willa Gelber, *A Feast for the Heart: Entertaining with Elegant and Easy Low-Cholesterol Menus* (Boston: Little, Brown, 1992).

Nancy Harmon Jenkins, *The Mediterranean Diet: A Delicious Alternative for Lifelong Health* (New York: Bantam, 1994).

Art Ulene, ed., *Count Out Cholesterol Cookbook: American Medical Association Campaign against Cholesterol* (New York: Knopf, 1989).

Obesity

National Academy Press
2101 Constitution Ave., N.W.
Washington, DC 20418
800-624-6242 (for orders)
Publication: *Weighing the Options: Critera for Evaluating Weight Management Programs*.

On the Internet: Two newsgroups, alt.support.big-folks and alt.support.obesity, provide online meeting places for people who are obese to share information.

Sandy Summers Head, *Sizing Up: Fashion, Fitness, and Self-Esteem for Full-Figured Women* (New York: Simon and Schuster, 1989).

Marvis Thompson and Kirk A. Johnson, *The Black Health Library Guide to Obesity* (New York: Holt, 1993).

Stroke

Michael Castleman, *An Aspirin a Day: What You Can Do to Prevent Heart Attack, Stroke, and Cancer* (New York: Hyperion, 1993).

Alcohol Use

American Council for Drug Education
136 E. 64th St.
New York, NY 10021
800-488-DRUG (800-488-3784)

National Clearinghouse for Alcohol and Drug Information
P.O. Box 2345
Rockville, MD 20847-2345
301-468-2600
800-729-6686

Diet

National Meals on Wheels
1133 20th St., N.W.
Washington, DC 20036
202-463-6039

Judith E. Brown, *Every Woman's Guide to Nutrition* (Minneapolis: University of Minnesota Press, 1991).

Elizabeth Somer, *Nutrition for Women: The Complete Guide* (New York: Henry Holt, 1993).

Estrogen Replacement Therapy

Susan M. Love and Karen Lindsey, *Dr. Susan Love's Hormone Book: Making Informed Choices about Menopause* (New York: Random House, 1997).

Lila Nachtigall and Joan R. Heilman, *Estrogen: A Complete Guide to Reversing the Effects of Menopause Using Hormone Replacement Therapy* (New York: HarperCollins, 1991).

Morris Notelovitz, *Estrogen: Yes or No?* (New York: St. Martin's Press, 1993).

Exercise

American Running and Fitness Association
9310 Georgetown Rd.
Bethesda, MD 20814
301-913-9517

Women's Sports Foundation
Suite 728
342 Madison Ave.
New York, NY 10173
800-227-3988

Elisabeth Bing and Libby Colman, *Losing Weight after Pregnancy: A Step-by-Step Guide to Postpartum Fitness* (New York: Hyperion, 1994).

Anne Kashiwa and James Rippe, *Fitness Walking for Women* (New York: Berkley, 1987).

Pat Lyons and Debby Burgard, *Great Shape: The First Fitness Guide for Large Women* (New York: Arbor/Morrow, 1988).

Melpolmene Institute for Women's Health Research, *The Bodywise Woman: Reliable Information about Physical Activity and Health* (Champaign, IL: Human Kinetics, 1993).

Smoking

American Cancer Society
800-ACS-2345
800-227-2345

Office on Smoking and Health
Mail Stop K-50
Atlanta, GA 30333
800-232-1311, Smoking, Tobacco, and Health
Information Line

On the Internet: A newsgroup, alt.support.stop-smoking, provides an on-line meeting place for people trying to kick the tobacco habit.

Harlan Krumholz and Robert Phillips, *No Ifs, Ands or Butts: The Smoker's Guide to Quitting* (Garden City, NY: Avery Publishing Group, 1993).

Stress Reduction

American Institute of Stress
124 Park Ave.
Yonkers, NY 10703
914-963-1200
800-24-RELAX (800-247-3529)
Publication: Newsletter; call for free sample.

Audiovision
3 Morningside Pl.
Norwalk, CT 06854
800-367-1604
Publication: Catalogue of books and audio and video tapes on managing stress, including "A Day Away from Stress" (available as audio or video), a combination of breathing exercises, guided imagery, music, and environmental sounds.

Harriet B. Braiker, *The Type E Woman: How to Overcome the Stress of Being Everything to Everybody* (New York: Signet, 1986).

David Elkind, *Ties That Stress: The New Family Imbalance* (Cambridge, MA: Harvard University Press, 1994).

Bonita C. Long and Sharon E. Kahn, *Women, Work, and Coping: A Multidisciplinary Approach to Workplace Stress* (Cheektowaga, NY: University of Toronto Press, 1993).

J. Robin Powell and Holly George-Warren, *The Working Woman's Guide to Managing Stress* (Needham Heights, MA: Prentice Hall School, 1994).

Weight Control

William I. Bennett and Joel Gurin, *Dieter's Dilemma* (New York: Basic Books, 1989).

Diane Epstein, *Feeding on Dreams: Why America's Diet Industry Doesn't Work and What Will Work for You* (New York: Macmillan, 1994).

Jane R. Hirschmann, *When Women Stop Hating Their Bodies: Freeing Yourself from Food and Weight Obsession* (New York: Fawcett, 1995).

Evelyn Tribole, *Intuitive Eating: A Recovery Book for the Chronic Dieter* (New York: St. Martin's, 1995).

Index